The Anti-Cancer Cookbook

Recipes to reduce your cancer risk

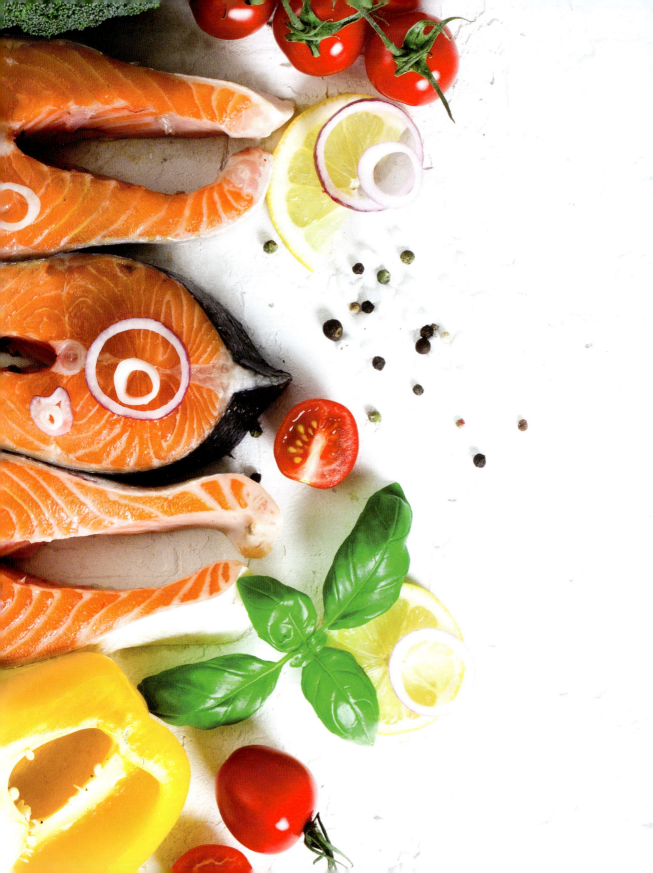

The Anti-Cancer Cookbook

Recipes to reduce your cancer risk

Dr Éadaoin Ní Bhuachalla PhD RD
Dr Aoife Ryan PhD RD

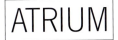

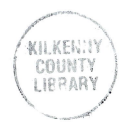

Foreword for
The Anti-Cancer Cookbook

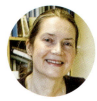 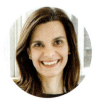 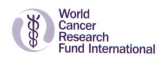

By Dr Kate Allen, Executive Director of Science & Public Affairs
Prof Martin Wiseman, Medical and Scientific Adviser
and Dr Giota Mitrou, Director of Research
World Cancer Research Fund

The recipes in this book are based on World Cancer Research Fund's (WCRF) 10 Cancer Prevention recommendations. To create these recommendations, WCRF reviewed and analysed decades of scientific research on diet, nutrition, physical activity and cancer – with the help of world-renowned, independent experts from across the globe. The sheer volume of evidence, the rigorous analysis, and the independent evaluation make these recommendations the most reliable advice available on diet, nutrition, and physical activity in relation to cancer prevention.

This huge repository of research, which we call the Continuous Update Project, strengthened the evidence that no one food or ingredient is important for cancer prevention. Instead, it is our diet and exercise patterns (and of course whether or not you smoke) across our whole life that makes us more or less susceptible to the mutations in cells that can lead to cancer.

That is why, for maximum benefit, our Cancer Prevention recommendations should be followed as a package of healthy behaviours – as they are the most reliable blueprint available for living healthily to reduce cancer risk. By following WCRF's Cancer Prevention recommendations, choosing not to smoke (or giving up smoking) and being safe when in the sun, you will have the best chance of living a life free from cancer. A growing number of studies in different countries and populations have shown that the more closely you follow WCRF's recommendations, the lower your risk of developing cancer; as well as of dying from cancer and other chronic diseases.

Cancer is the second leading cause of death globally. As more countries adopt 'Western' lifestyles – that is diets with large amounts of highly processed foods, with a mostly sedentary pattern of behaviour – the number of new cases of cancer is expected to rise from 18 million globally in 2018, to 30 million by 2040. That is why evidence-based health advice for cancer prevention is invaluable, as around 40% of cancers could be prevented if people were healthier; that includes maintaining a healthy weight by being active and eating a healthy diet, and not smoking.

> ## *An ounce of prevention is worth a pound of cure*
>
> Benjamin Franklin

Patients who have been given the bad news of a cancer diagnosis often ask, 'What did I do to deserve this? What did I do wrong? Could I have avoided this?' Those who have tried to lead healthy lives often feel particularly disappointed and indeed cheated that their efforts have not been more justly rewarded.

It is hard for people in this difficult situation to understand that there usually isn't a single recognisable cause for an individual patient's cancer. It is often just bad luck. How can this be?

Every day in our bodies, millions of our cells divide, forming 'daughter' cells. This process is normal, and usually works well, but every now and then the division is faulty and one of the cells is left with an abnormality called a 'mutation'. Many mutant cells simply die off, with no health consequences. Others survive, and pass on their mutations to their own daughter cells, which can in turn suffer additional mutations. Over our lives this process occurs many times, and sometimes, if a cell survives enough of these and accumulates enough mutations, it becomes a 'cancer cell'.

We have some control over the development of mutations in our bodies, mostly by avoiding very dangerous 'mutation-causing' behaviours. Smoking provides the most obvious example. Tobacco smoke bathes the mouth, lungs and throat with 'carcinogenic', i.e. cancer-causing, chemicals. Other tobacco carcinogens get into the bloodstream and can predispose to cancers of the bladder, pancreas and other organs. The advice on smoking is simple. Don't start. If you smoke – give up.

It is obvious that our diets can also affect our health. We are, after all, what we eat. While it is generally understood by the public that diet is centrally incriminated in causing diabetes and circulatory diseases, the influence of diet on cancer is less widely understood. The information available to the public in this regard is often ill-informed and misleading. The frequency with which the lay press warns against specific cancer-causing foods seems to be rivalled only by their enthusiasm for endorsing alleged cancer-preventing 'super-foods' and supplements. As is pointed out by the authors of *The Anti-Cancer Cookbook,* many of these reports are highly inaccurate, and are in some cases frankly dangerous.

So what is the truth about diet and cancer? Dietary practices also have clearly been shown to influence the chance of developing mutations and ultimately cancer. However, unlike smoking, we do have to eat.

One of the most important observations in this book is that the biggest potential cancer benefit from dietary modification comes not from eliminating bad foods, but from reducing calorie intake in general, regardless of the source. Obesity, no matter how it originates, is a definite cause of cancer, and as such we probably need to concentrate on eating less, rather than on avoiding specific cancer-causing foods. This has been reinforced by recent research which has highlighted the fact that, for some cancers, obesity is a bigger culprit than smoking. Examples include cancers of the kidney, bowel, womb and liver. The increases in these cancers associated with obesity are typically in the 20–30% range (in contrast to smoking, where lung cancer increases the risk by several multiples).

In *The Anti-Cancer Cookbook*, the authors do an excellent job of explaining these subtleties. They outline the impact of diet and provide sensible, data-based advice on how to reduce our cancer risk without taking all the pleasure out of eating, by following simple, realistic and very achievable recommendations. The scientific validity of their recommendations is rivalled only by the healthy, tasty recipes which they include.

Sláinte and Bon Appétit!

Professor John Crown
Consultant Medical Oncologist,
St Vincent's University Hospital
Dublin

Endorsements and Testimonials

'In a world where there are so many mixed messages about what to eat (and what not to eat) it is wonderful to have this well-researched book to help patients, families and the general public make better decisions to improve their diet and their health. Well done to the authors who continue to provide us with these resources to contribute to better nutritional health for everyone'.

Jennifer Feighan, CEO, Irish Nutrition & Dietetic Institute

'A really fantastic book. The recipes look great and very appetising (not to mention healthy!)'.

Louise Reynolds, Communications Manager, Irish Nutrition & Dietetic Institute

'Since losing my mum to cancer and becoming a dad to my beautiful twins, I have a new appreciation of health and nutrition. It is so important to recognise that eating well really helps our overall wellbeing, our mental health and can help prevent cancer'.

Neven Maguire, Chef and Author

'A truly superb book addressing the ever-important issue of cancer prevention. With one in every three cancers thought to be preventable, this book is for the entire population. My congratulations to the authors for bringing the scientific information down to everyday healthy meals suitable for the entire family'.

Dr Derek Power, Consultant Medical Oncologist, Cork & Mercy University Hospitals, Ireland

'The Anti-Cancer Cookbook is the exact nutritional resource that I would have loved to have had available to me pre, during and post cancer treatment. An evidence based guide from nutritional scientific experts along with easy to prepare tasty and healthful recipes. The Anti-Cancer Cookbook is a welcome antidote to the abundance of potentially harmful fad diets and misinformation around the topic of cancer and diet'.

Ms Eileen O'Sullivan, Cancer Patient Advocate

'This book transforms some of the best scientific research in the world into a delicious guide on how healthy eating can help protect against diet-related cancers. The authors explain how different foods bring different benefits. This book will empower people touched by cancer because it provides information that can be trusted on how to make the most out of our health from the food we eat'.

Dr Mary A.T. Flynn RD, Chief Specialist Public Health Nutrition, Food Safety Authority of Ireland and Visiting Professor, Ulster University, Coleraine, Northern Ireland

'Food is central to cancer treatment and prevention. This cook book is instrumental in bringing whole grains, fruits and vegetables to the centre of the plate, consistent with the American Institute for Cancer Research official recognition that the majority of foods on a plate need to be of plant origin. This book plays a role in solidifying the burgeoning awareness that fresh, wholesome plant foods (as compared to industrially processed foods sold in supermarkets or meat-central meals) are health-promoting. The lush pictures of the dishes provide excitement to try these simple, yet novel and reliable recipes!'

Prof Niyati Parekh, Cancer Epidemiologist, Associate Professor of Public Health Nutrition, New York University

Contents

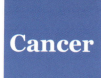

Cancer

Cancer causes one in six deaths worldwide and has overtaken cardiovascular disease as the leading cause of death in many parts of the world. There were 17 million new cases of cancer and 9.6 million deaths from cancer in 2018 and this global cancer burden is expected to increase to 27.5 million new cases per year by 2040.

What is cancer?

Every part of our body is made up of small units called cells. These cells are constantly growing, dividing, dying off and being replaced. This cycle is essential for the human body to function and is very tightly controlled by DNA in healthy individuals. Cancer occurs when our DNA becomes damaged and the body's cells divide and multiply without control. Cancer cells rapidly split and copy themselves, which results in many new cancer cells being formed. This uncontrollable growth causes cancer cells to spread to other parts of the body. These cells do not die off as normal cells do, and eventually these accumulating cancer cells form lumps or tumours. Cancer can occur anywhere in the body and there are many different forms. Each type of cancer will have a unique effect on the body and will cause different symptoms in different people.

What causes cancer?

Cancer occurs when our DNA, which controls how our cells grow and divide, becomes damaged. Some people inherit damaged DNA from their parents; however, the majority of DNA damage occurs during our lifetime. Although people often believe getting cancer is down to genes, fate or bad luck, the reality is the vast majority of cancers are caused by things we come in contact with in our environment during our lives. Scientists estimate that 2-3 cases of cancer in 100 are due to inherited genes, while between 20 and 50 per cent of all cancer cases are estimated to be preventable.

Things that promote cancer development are also known as carcinogens. Carcinogens have different levels of cancer-causing potential and do not cause cancer in every person. The risk of developing cancer depends on numerous factors including a person's genetic make-up, as well as the length and intensity of carcinogen exposure. Trying to pin down the cause of any cancer is impossible and the development of the disease is not straightforward or attributable to a single risk factor. There are no quick fixes or magic ingredients that will mean you won't develop cancer. However, we know that **there are a number of modifiable factors that increase the risk of cancer and therefore making healthier lifestyle choices can tangibly reduce the risk of developing the disease.**

Not smoking or using any form of tobacco, and avoiding other exposure to tobacco smoke, are the most important means of reducing cancer risk.

The next most important means of reducing risk (and the most important for non-smokers) is to maintain a healthy weight throughout life by consuming a healthy diet and being physically active. Other risk factors include long-term infections, radiation, sun exposure and tanning and industrial chemicals. Minimising exposure to these risk factors is another means of reducing cancer risk.

Is cancer preventable?

> **'Avoidance of tobacco in any form, together with appropriate diet and nutrition, physical activity and maintaining a healthy weight, have the potential over time to reduce much of the global burden of cancer'**

Although a number of factors that alter cancer risk are out of our control (e.g. age, gender) there is still much we can do to decrease our risk. It is now well accepted by the scientific community that over one third of the world's most common cancers could be preventable through a number of lifestyle changes. These mainly involve avoidance of smoking, maintaining a healthy body weight, eating a healthy diet, reducing alcohol consumption, keeping active, being sun safe, and doing what you can to avoid certain cancer-causing infections. Looking specifically at the influence of body weight, nutrition and physical activity, research has shown that 67% of cancers of the mouth and throat, 45% of bowel cancers, 44% of womb cancers, 38% of breast cancers, 33% of lung cancers, 34% of oesophageal (food pipe/gullet) cancers, 15–29% of cancers of the pancreas, gallbladder, stomach, liver and kidney are preventable through the maintenance of a healthy body weight, a healthy diet and regular exercise.

The purpose of this book is not to blame people for their cancer or to tell people what they have done wrong. Cancer prevention is not a guarantee. The aim is to help people understand what cancer is, what causes it and what steps can be taken to **reduce** your risk of developing cancer. There is a wealth of scientific evidence available that highlights the associations between lifestyle and cancer risk; however, research has also shown that people are unaware of the evidence or misinformed in terms of what truly influences cancer risk. The main objective of this resource is to make people aware of the evidence and to give them the tools to make healthy changes to their lifestyle in order to promote cancer prevention. Any change, big or small, made from now on will make a difference and help to stack the odds in your favour.

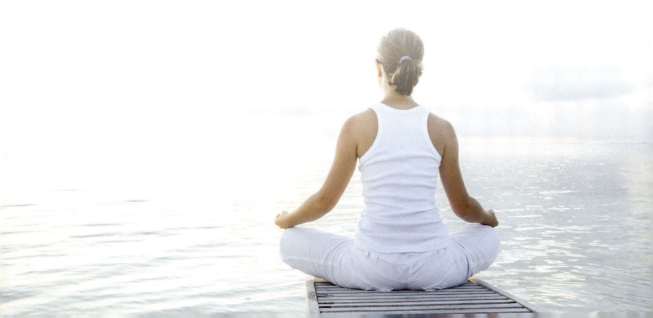

How can I reduce the risk of getting cancer?

There are thousands of websites, books, blogs, articles and experts giving advice on how best to prevent cancer. This makes it very difficult to distinguish fact from fiction. The most reliable information from all of the scientific studies that have been performed are the expert reports published by the World Cancer Research Fund (WCRF) and the American Institute for Cancer Research (AICR). These reports are endorsed by the World Health Organisation and many other international organisations. Panels of expert scientists review the scientific evidence from hundreds and thousands of scientific papers.

The latest cancer prevention recommendations come from the WCRF's Expert Report (2018) and from the conclusions of an independent panel of experts. The recommendations represent a package of healthy lifestyle choices which together can make an enormous impact on people's likelihood of developing cancer and other noncommunicable diseases over their lifetimes.

The key recommendations for cancer prevention in the 2018 report are as follows:

- Be a healthy weight – keep your weight within the healthy range and avoid weight gain in adult life (page 10)
- Be physically active as part of everyday life – walk more and sit less (page 12)
- Eat wholegrains, vegetables, fruit and beans – make these part of your usual diet (page 15)
- Limit consumption of 'fast foods' – and other processed foods high in fat, starches or sugars (page 20)
- Limit red and processed meat – eat no more than moderate amounts of red meat, such as beef, pork and lamb
- Eat little, if any, processed meat (page 23)
- Limit sugar-sweetened drinks – drink mostly water and unsweetened drinks (page 26)
- Limit alcohol consumption – for cancer prevention, it's best not to drink alcohol (page 28)
- Don't rely on supplements – aim to meet nutritional needs through diet alone (page 31)
- Breastfeed your baby, if you can – breastfeeding is good for both mother and baby (page 33)
- After a cancer diagnosis, follow these recommendations if you can (page 36)

The Expert Panel from the WCRF emphasise in their most recent 2018 report the importance of recognising that, 'while following each individual recommendation is expected to offer cancer protection, the most benefit is to be gained by treating them as an integrated pattern of behaviours relating to diet and physical activity, and other factors, that can be considered as a single overarching "package" or way of life'.

Can these lifestyle changes really make a difference?

Yes, and not just for cancer. As already mentioned, cancer prevention is not a guarantee. However, research has been performed in huge numbers of people and has shown that overall, when the average person follows the WCRF cancer prevention guidelines, a reduction in cancer risk is seen.

One of the largest studies that has been performed to date is the European Prospective Investigation into Cancer and Nutrition study, or 'EPIC' study, which includes over 380,000 people. This study followed people for over 10 years and looked at their adherence to the cancer prevention recommendations made by the WCRF and whether people developed cancer. The study found that for every WCRF recommendation that a person complied with, they had a 5% lower chance of getting cancer. **People that had the best compliance with the guidelines had lower**

risk of cancer and a 34% lower risk of death overall, compared to those that had poor compliance with the recommendations. In terms of specific cancers, complying with more than 5 of the WCRF recommendations significantly reduced people's risk as follows: lung (14%), liver (15%), breast (16%), endometrial (23%), colorectal (27%), kidney (29%), upper aero-digestive tract (31%), stomach (38%) and oesophageal (food pipe/gullet) cancer (42%) (Romaguera et al., 2012).

Studies have also shown the effect the guidelines have on the risk of cancer death and risk of death from any cause. A recent study of over 16,000 people looked at those that adhered to few of the guidelines compared to those that adhered to most of the guidelines. The scientists found that those that did not follow guidelines had an 18% higher risk of death from any cause. In terms of cancer deaths, there was higher risk of death from the following cancers in both men and women that had poor adherence to the WCRF guidelines: lung (28% increased risk), head and neck cancers (51% increased risk), stomach (66% increased risk) and prostate (men only) (52% increased risk) (Lohse et al., 2016).

There are also wider benefits of cancer prevention – trends in other non-communicable diseases (NCDs) including diabetes, chronic respiratory disease and cardiovascular disease show that these all share common underlying risk factors including diet, obesity, physical inactivity, alcohol consumption, tobacco use and certain long-term infections. Therefore approaches to preventing cancer can provide benefits across a range of NCDs.

Who is this book for?

This book is for healthy people who would like to reduce their risk of cancer. Patients with cancer should receive nutritional care from an appropriately trained individual (ideally a registered dietician). If able to do so, and unless otherwise advised, cancer survivors should aim to follow the recommendations for cancer prevention. If people have been diagnosed with an illness, they should consult with their doctor or registered dietitian to check what is suitable for them before altering their lifestyle.

It is important to make realistic changes. This book goes through each of the ten diet and lifestyle recommendations made by the WCRF, judge which one is most realistic for you and start with that. Implement additional changes once you have incorporated the other changes into your lifestyle. Trying to change too much at once is difficult to maintain and we want to help you to make these changes for life.

Recommendation 1

Be a healthy weight.

Keep your weight within the healthy range and avoid weight gain in adult life.

There is strong evidence that greater body fatness causes many cancers, and this evidence has strengthened over the last 10 years. The risk is higher the more weight a person gains and the longer they are overweight for. **Maintaining a healthy body weight throughout life is one of the most important ways to protect against cancer.**

There is now 'convincing' scientific evidence that being overweight or obese throughout adulthood increases the risk of: mouth, pharynx and larynx cancers, oesophageal cancer (adenocarcinoma), stomach cancer (cardia), pancreatic cancer, liver cancer, colorectal cancer, breast cancer (postmenopausal), ovarian cancer, endometrial cancer (cancer of the womb), prostate cancer (advanced) and kidney cancer. Greater weight gain in adulthood increases the risk of postmenopausal breast cancer.

Body fatness is difficult to measure directly without special equipment. Body Mass Index (BMI) is commonly used as a measure of weight in relation to your height. BMI is calculated as weight in kilograms divided by height in metres squared (kg/m^2). BMI charts and calculators are available online that can be easily used to classify your weight for height score. It is recommended that individuals keep their BMI within a healthy range. The World Health Organisation (WHO) have classified healthy or 'normal' weight adults as having a BMI of $18.5-24.9 kg/m^2$, underweight as $<18.5 kg/m^2$, overweight as $25-29.9 kg/m^2$, and obese as $>30 kg/m^2$.

Where fat is stored in the body is also important. Storing fat around the abdomen (or belly) is commonly referred to as an 'apple shape'. Excess abdominal/belly fat is a cause of a number of chronic diseases including Type 2 diabetes, cardiovascular disease and many cancers.

Being overweight doesn't mean that someone will definitely develop cancer. But if a person is overweight they are more likely to get cancer than if they are a healthy weight. Consistent results from decades of research involving millions of people show the strong link between obesity and cancer and mean we can confidently rule out other reasons (such as chance or other lifestyle factors). The risk increases the more weight is gained.

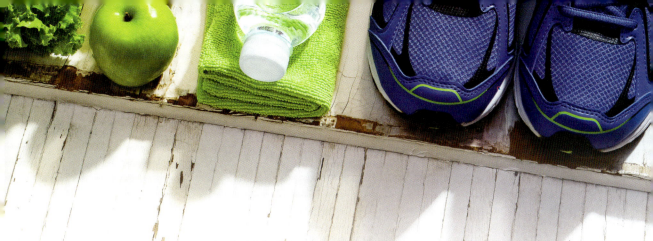

There are many reasons why extra body fat is linked with cancer. For some cancers like oesophageal cancer, increased body fatness may promote acid reflux which may lead to damage or inflammation of the oesophagus, which over time can increase the risk of oesophageal cancer. For colorectal cancer, high body fatness is associated with changes in hormonal profiles, such as increased levels of insulin, which can promote the growth of colon cancer cells and prevent the body's own natural way of killing off damaged cells. Higher levels of insulin and higher levels of inflammatory proteins in the blood as a result of obesity can also promote the development of many cancers including colorectal and postmenopausal breast cancer. In postmenopausal women with increased body fatness, higher levels of hormones like insulin and oestrogen (made in fat tissue) are in the blood. These are only a few examples of the role excess body weight can play in cancer development.

What can I do to maintain a healthy weight and lifestyle?

The best advice for maintaining a healthy weight is to be physically active, consume a diet rich in wholegrains, fruit and vegetables, and limit the consumption of sugar-sweetened drinks and energy-dense foods (convenience foods) that are high in fat, sugar and salt.

Plant foods are generally low in energy (with a few exceptions) and eating a large amount of plant food helps to control the amount of food and calories (energy) we consume. This in turn helps to prevent excess weight gain. Fruit and vegetables also form an important part of the diet to prevent against cancer development. It is best to choose whole, fresh fruit and vegetables, rather than processed or tinned foods that are high in sugar or salt. Red meat should be consumed in low to moderate amounts and processed meat should be avoided. Alcoholic drinks should also be consumed in small amounts, if at all. Alcohol is very high in energy (calories) and has been shown to be linked to many cancers.

Being physically active daily helps to maintain a healthy weight, as well as improving cardiovascular fitness. It is recommended that individuals be physically active for at least 30 minutes every day. As fitness improves, this should be increased to 60 minutes or 30 minutes of vigorous activity, equating to approximately 150 minutes per week. Even standing up or getting up and about at work can help to increase the amount of time spent being active.

Recommendation 2

Be Physically Active.

Be physically active for at least 30 minutes every day.

PERSONAL RECOMMENDATIONS

- Be moderately physically active, equivalent to brisk walking, for at least 30 minutes every day.
- As fitness improves, aim for 60 minutes or more of moderate, or 30 minutes or more of vigorous, physical activity every day.
- Limit sedentary habits such as watching television.

Physical activity improves the health of everyone, no matter what age. The benefits of being physically active range from disease prevention to improved mental health and much more. People who do not achieve recommended levels of physical activity have a 20–30% higher risk of death compared to those who are active. Physical inactivity is the fourth leading cause of death worldwide. Physical activity has been proven to reduce the risk of many diseases including cancer, heart disease, stroke and diabetes. It helps to burn off energy/calories from food and therefore is essential for preventing overweight or obesity. The more exercise we do, the greater the health benefits.

How does physical activity affect cancer risk?

Physical activity helps to reduce cancer risk in a number of ways. Moderate to vigorous activity has been shown to directly reduce the risk of breast, bowel and womb cancer. In addition, regular physical activity can prevent weight gain, overweight and obesity and therefore helps to prevent the development of obesity-related cancers.

Physical activity also helps to reduce inflammation (inflammation promotes cancer growth), and improves immune function. It also helps with the production of healthy levels of hormones in the body. In some cancer sites, physical activity has a direct impact. For example, physical activity aids the bowel by encouraging regular bowel movements. This reduces the amount of time waste takes to pass through the gut, reducing the bowel's exposure to toxins, which in turn reduces the risk of bowel cancer.

Are certain forms of exercise better than others?

The evidence linking physical activity to cancer risk is based on moderate to vigorous aerobic activity. Moderate activity includes any exercise that makes your heart beat faster and increases your breathing but you can still maintain a conversation. You will be warm and produce a light sweat, e.g. brisk walk (1 mile in 15–20 minutes), jogging (a mile in >10 minutes), cycling (< 10 miles per hour), medium-paced swimming, ballroom dancing, general gardening.

Vigorous exercise causes heavy breathing, with a faster heart rate and more sweating. It would be a struggle to keep a conversation going while exercising vigorously. Examples of vigorous activity include: jogging/running (1 mile in <10 minutes); fast cycling (>10 miles per hour); active sports such as hurling, football, soccer, basketball, squash or aerobics; circuit training; swimming lengths; fast-paced dancing such as salsa, Irish dancing, quick step, etc; skipping; heavy gardening; or hill-walking with a backpack.

It is best to include a mixture of moderate and vigorous activity over the week. In addition it is advisable to also include activities that increase muscle strength, balance and flexibility. Muscle strengthening activities help to keep your muscles strong and this helps you to carry out your daily activities. Having more muscle and stronger muscle is really beneficial as you get older, helping you to remain independent, and it is also really import for recovery from illness, surgery or some medical treatments, e.g. surgery, chemotherapy, radiotherapy. Strength exercise includes using hand-held weights, weight machines or using your body weight to build muscle. Exercises to improve balance and flexibility help to prevent falls and to keep your muscles limber. These include: stretches, standing from sitting, standing on one foot, walking on heels and toes, yoga and tai chi.

It is also important to remember that physical activity doesn't just have to be performed during your leisure time. Physical activity includes the exercise involved in transport (e.g. walking or cycling to work, school or college), occupation (jobs that include activity or manual labour), as well as recreational activities.

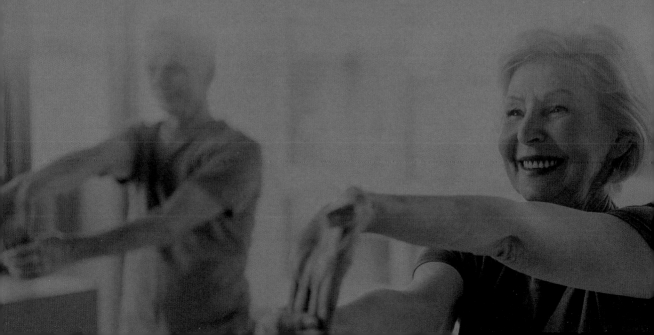

How much exercise should I be doing?

First and foremost, you should always exercise as tolerated and gradually build up your exercise levels at a comfortable rate. If you have chronic conditions such as diabetes, heart disease or osteoarthritis, a lack of mobility, or experience chest pain, dizziness or joint pain, you should speak with your doctor before increasing your physical activity levels and look for advice on how to include physical activity safely. Even if you are limited in what exercise you can do, you should aim to be as active as you are able to be.

It is recommended that at a minimum, adults should engage in 30 minutes of moderate activity 5 days a week. Exercise can be broken up into shorter bouts, but these need to last longer than 10 minutes.

Engaging in vigorous activity is roughly equal to twice the amount of moderate activity, so 75 minutes of vigorous activity would meet recommendations as it is equivalent to 150 minutes of moderate activity. It is best to spread exercise out over the week and to include a variety of exercise types.

This is recommended as the minimum level of physical activity, and greater health benefits are yielded from increased exercise. It is optimal to include at least 60 minutes of moderate activity on 5 days of the week, totalling 300 minutes (or 150 minutes of vigorous activity). Again, it's best to spread this out over the week and to include different forms of exercise to yield maximum benefits.

Limiting sedentary habits

Sedentary is another word for being inactive. Being sedentary means that your body is not doing any work and usually involves sitting or lying down for a period of time. There is convincing evidence that the more time you spend sedentary, the greater the risk of developing cancer. Sedentary activities include watching television, computer work, using your smartphone or driving.

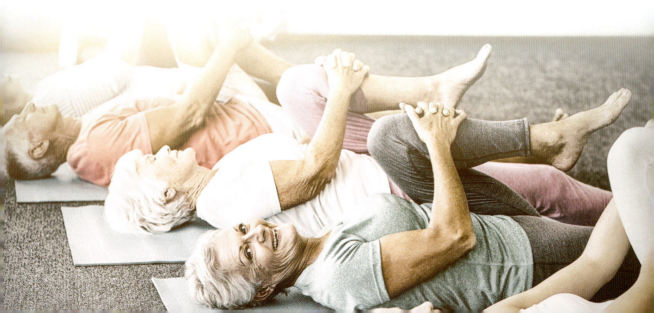

Recommendation 3

Eat a diet rich in wholegrains, vegetables, fruit and beans.

PERSONAL RECOMMENDATIONS

- Consume a diet that provides at least 30g per day of fibre from food sources.
- Eat a diet high in all types of plant foods including at least 5 portions or servings (at least 400g or 14oz in total) of a variety of non-starchy vegetables and fruit every day.
- Include in most meals foods containing wholegrains, non-starchy vegetables, fruit, and pulses (legumes) such as beans and lentils.

There is strong scientific evidence that eating wholegrains protects against colorectal cancer, and that eating foods containing dietary fibre protects against colorectal cancer and against weight gain, overweight and obesity. Most diets that are protective against cancer are rich in foods of plant origin.

What is a plant food?

Plant foods are foods that are derived from plants and are naturally high in nutrients, high in dietary fibre but low in energy density. Our diets should be based primarily on plant foods, particularly unprocessed cereals and grains, non-starchy vegetables and fruit, legumes and pulses (peas, beans and lentils), with a limited amount of food derived from animals, e.g. meat products, dairy products. Examples of plant foods include fruit, vegetables, wholegrains and legumes. One portion of non-starchy vegetables or fruit is approximately 80g or 3oz.

Unprocessed cereals and grains

Cereals (grains) are the seeds of cultivated grasses, e.g. wheat, rice, maize (corn), millet, barley, oats and rye. The majority of the cereals and grains that we eat are processed or refined. During manufacturing, the grains are broken up into pieces and different parts of the grain are sifted out to produce a grain that is easier to chew, faster to cook and lighter in colour, e.g. white rice, white flour. A lot of the fibre, protein and B vitamins in the original grain are lost through this processing or refining. Grains commonly go through additional processing before they reach the supermarket shelf, e.g. the addition of sugar to cereals during the production of processed breakfast cereals. On the other hand, wholegrain products go through limited processing and generally the grain is kept intact. In this way unprocessed grains (wholegrains) are a much better source of nutrition, providing more dietary fibre, resistant starch, antioxidants and vitamins and minerals. Examples of foods that contain unprocessed cereals and grains include brown rice, oats, brown pasta, wholegrain or brown bread, quinoa and unsweetened breakfast cereals.

Non-starchy vegetables

Vegetables can be categorised into two main groups: non-starchy and starchy vegetables. Starchy vegetables include potatoes, yam, sweet potatoes and plantain. Although they are classified as vegetables by some, they are high in carbohydrate and therefore they do not count towards your fruit and vegetable intake. Instead they are counted as a carbohydrate source, i.e. an alternative to pasta, rice or bread in the diet.

Non-starchy vegetables count towards your fruit and vegetable intake and are a rich source of vitamins, minerals and fibre. Non-starchy vegetables can be further divided into different families including green, leafy vegetables (e.g. spinach, lettuce, kale), root vegetables (carrots, butternut squash, beets, parsnips, turnips, swedes), cruciferous vegetables (the cabbage family, e.g. cabbage, brussels sprouts, broccoli, cauliflower) and allium vegetables (e.g. onions, garlic and leeks).

Legumes and pulses

Legumes are a family of plant foods which include fresh peas, fresh beans, soybeans, peanuts and pulses. Pulses refer to the dried seed of the legume family and include foods such as dried peas, chickpeas, beans and lentils. Legumes have an important role in the cancer prevention diet as they are plant foods that are both high in protein and a rich source of fibre, therefore providing a nutritious alternative to meat.

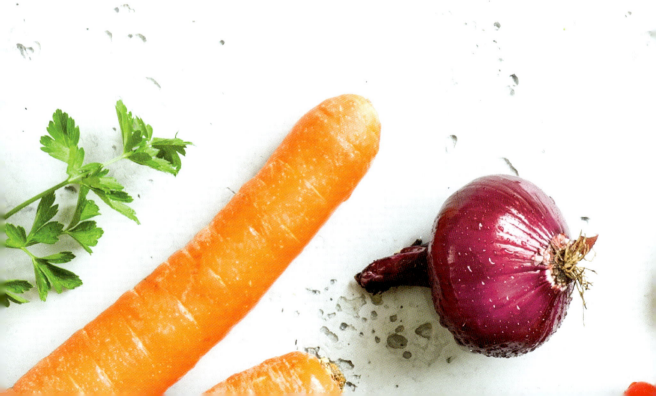

How do plant foods alter cancer risk?

Plant foods reduce cancer risk in three main ways.

The strongest evidence linking plant foods and cancer is for fibre-containing plant foods (e.g. fruit, vegetables, wholegrain bread, wholegrain rice, brown pasta, oats) and bowel cancer. Fibre has many different benefits, one of the main ones being helping to maintain regular bowel movements. Fibre helps to speed up the passage of food through our gut, something which is thought to be beneficial for cancer prevention, particularly for cancers of the bowel. A review of all the studies looking at fibre and bowel cancer found that for every 10g of fibre eaten every day, there is a 10% lower risk of developing bowel cancer. Getting fibre by eating legumes showed the best risk reduction (e.g. peas, beans, chickpeas, lentils) (38% reduced risk of cancer), followed by eating wholegrain cereals, fruit and vegetables (WCRF/AICR Systematic Literature Review Continuous Update Project Report, Colorectal Cancer 2010).

Individual groups of fruits and vegetables have also been shown to reduce the risk of specific cancers. There is strong evidence to show that eating non-starchy vegetables protects against cancers of the mouth and throat. There is strong evidence to show that garlic is protective against cancers of the bowel. Higher fruit consumption is protective against cancers of the mouth, throat and lung. Fruit and vegetables are rich sources of vitamins and minerals, which help to keep our immune system and our body healthy; they are also good sources of phytochemicals and antioxidants. These compounds are very active and can help to protect our bodies from damage to cells which can lead to cancer.

Finally, plant foods are generally low in energy/calories (with a few exceptions) and eating a large amount of plant food helps to control the number of calories we consume. Therefore consuming plant foods helps us to achieve the first cancer prevention recommendation of maintaining a healthy body weight and preventing overweight/obesity, something which we know is associated with an increased risk of 12 different cancers.

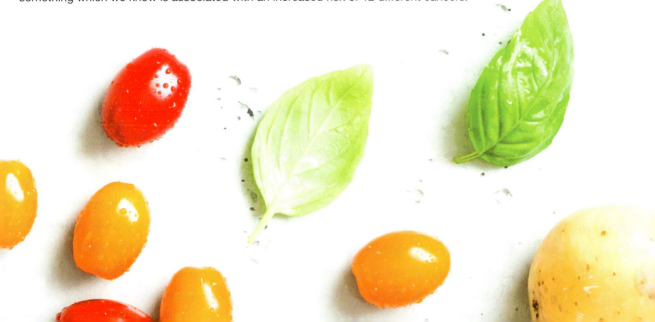

Which 'plant foods' should I be eating and how much?

Plant food should make up the majority of our diet, with a limited amount of animal foods. The WCRF recommends eating at least 400g (14oz) of fruit and non-starchy vegetables a day, which equates to a minimum of 5 portions or '5-a-day'. Fresh, frozen, dried and canned in water or natural juices all count towards your '5 a day'. Limit fruit juice to unsweetened varieties and only one glass a day. Limit dried fruit to 1 tablespoon a day (30g). Pulses, e.g. lentils, peas and beans, also count towards 1 portion of your '5-a-day' and are also a great source of fibre and protein.

Different types of fruit and vegetables contain different vitamins, minerals and phytochemicals and that is why including a variety of these foods is so important. A good rule of thumb is to include a range of different-coloured fruit and vegetables in your daily diet. This will help to ensure you are eating a range of different vitamins and minerals.

One portion of fruit and vegetables is roughly 80g weighed ($2^1/_2$ – 3 oz). Examples of 1 serving are listed below:

- 3 heaped tablespoons of cooked vegetables, e.g. carrots, parsnips, broccoli
- 1 cereal bowl of salad leaves, e.g. lettuce, rocket
- 1 slice of a large fruit, e.g. melon
- 1 medium whole fruit, e.g. apple, banana, orange
- 2 small whole fruits, e.g. plums, kiwis, mandarin orange
- 1–2 handfuls of berries, e.g. strawberries, raspberries, blueberries
- 3–4 heaped tablespoons of cooked or canned pulses, e.g. beans, peas or lentils
- 1 tablespoon of dried pulses, e.g. dried lentils, dried chickpeas

Starchy vegetables (e.g. potatoes, sweet potatoes, yam), grains (e.g. rice, quinoa or oats) and anything fruit flavoured (or containing added sugar or salt) (e.g. fruit jams, olives) do not count towards your 5-a-day.

Aside from fruit, vegetables and pulses, our plate should contain healthy grains and cereals, e.g. rice, oats, pasta, bread, couscous and unsweetened breakfast cereal. We should always choose wholegrain or brown varieties over 'white'. It is important to limit processed grains and cereals, as these can be high in fat, sugar and salt.

As a rule of thumb, at mealtimes a minimum of three-quarters of our plate should be made up of wholegrains, fruit, vegetables and pulses. The remaining quarter (or less) should contain lean meats, fish or other protein foods. Please see the infographic on the opposite page as an example of how your plate should look at mealtimes. Meat has traditionally been the centre of Irish meals; however, we need to rethink the way we plan our meals and start centring our dishes on plant foods rather than animal foods. This change will greatly help to reduce our risk of many different cancers and will reduce overweight/obesity.

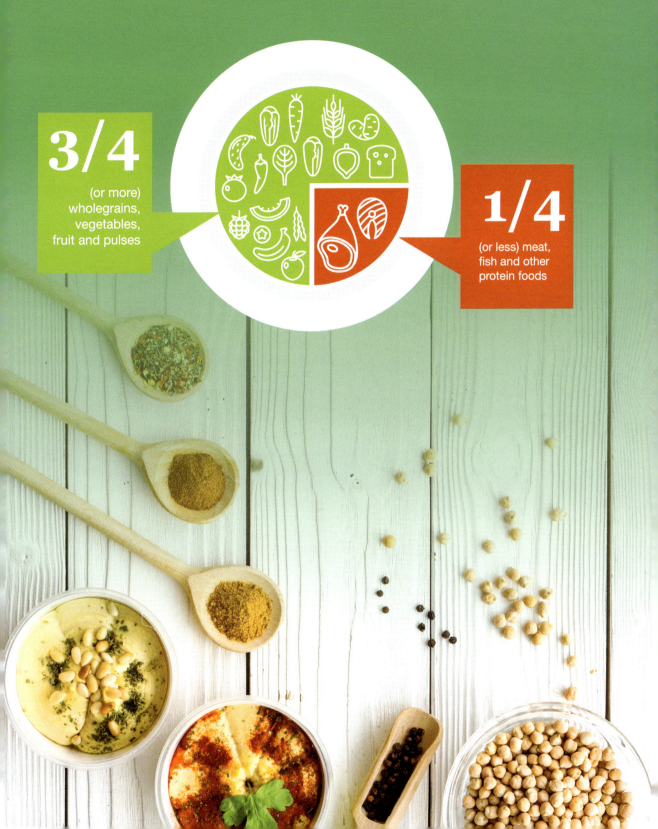

3/4

(or more)
wholegrains,
vegetables,
fruit and pulses

1/4

(or less) meat,
fish and other
protein foods

Recommendation 4

Limit consumption of 'fast foods' and other processed foods high in fat, starches or sugars.

Limiting these foods helps control calorie intake and maintain a healthy weight.

There is strong evidence that diets containing greater amounts of 'fast foods' and other processed foods that are high in fat, starches or sugars are a cause of excess weight gain and obesity. These foods are generally highly palatable, high in energy, cheap, easy to access and easy to store. As a result these foods have been shown to contribute to excess intake of energy/calories and lead to weight gain. There is strong evidence that greater body fatness is a cause of many cancers.

What is energy density?

Energy density measures the amount of energy (or calories) a food supplies in a given weight of the food (usually 100g). If a food has a high energy density it means it provides a large amount of calories in a small volume of the food, e.g. confectionery, fast food. On the other hand, a food that is low in energy density provides a small amount of calories in a large amount of the food, e.g. fruit, vegetables.

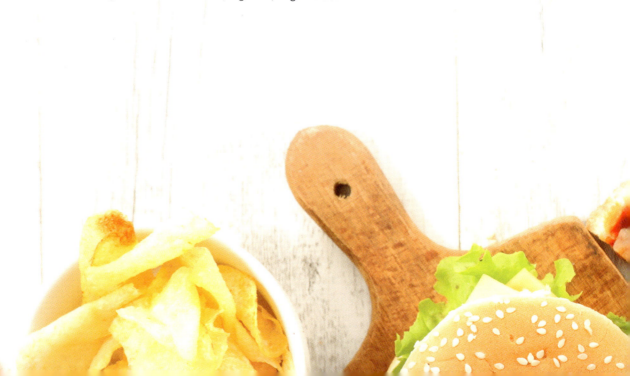

How will I know whether a food is energy dense?

As a general rule, processed foods that contain lots of fat/sugar and little fibre tend to have a high energy density, whereas fresh foods that are not processed tend to have a lower energy density. There are some whole foods that are naturally energy dense (e.g. nuts, seeds), however when these are consumed in moderation as part of a healthy balanced diet they have not been associated with weight gain or an increased risk of cancer, and are often a valuable source of nutrients.

Most foods display nutritional information on their labels and usually list how many calories (kcal) the food contains per 100g of food. The following categorisation will then allow you to check whether the foods have a low, moderate or high energy density.

AMOUNT OF ENERGY (CALORIES) IN 100G OF FOOD		
HIGH ENERGY DENSITY	**MEDIUM ENERGY DENSITY**	**LOW ENERGY DENSITY**
Over 225 calories (kcal)	125–225 calories (kcal)	<125 calories (kcal)
E.g. fast foods, cakes, biscuits, crisps, confectionery, butter and other spreads.	E.g. bread, cooked brown pasta, cooked brown rice, lean meat, poultry and fish.	E.g. most vegetables, fruits and cooked pulses.

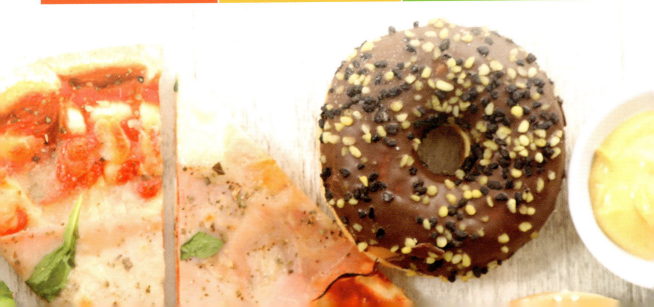

How do energy-dense foods affect cancer risk?

Foods and diets that have a high energy density cause weight gain and promote overweight and obesity. The primary goal of this recommendation is to help us to achieve the first recommendation of maintaining a healthy body weight, because overweight and obesity are strong risk factors for cancer.

Aside from weight gain, energy density is also an important measure of the quality of the diet. Foods that are high in energy density generally have a poor nutritional quality. By avoiding energy-dense foods, the diet will naturally be low in processed foods and high in plant-based foods, two cornerstones of cancer prevention and healthy-eating diets.

What is considered a 'sugary drink' and why should we avoid them?

Sugary drinks refer to drinks with added sugar, e.g. sugar-sweetened fizzy drinks and juices with added sugar. Sugary drinks provide a lot of calories but do not provide any nutritional value and do not make us feel full. In this way they lead to overconsumption of calories and lead to weight gain. (See page 26 for more information.)

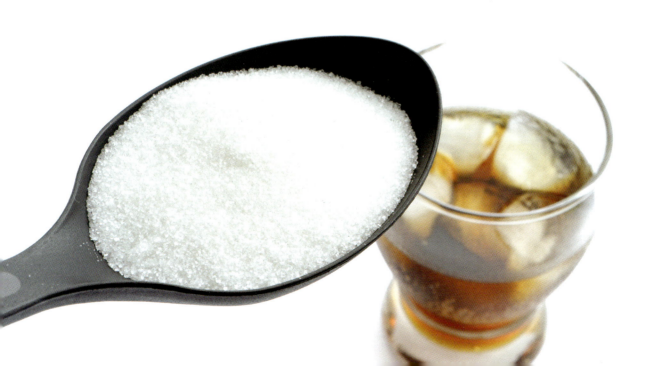

Recommendation 5

Limit consumption of red meat and processed meat.

PERSONAL RECOMMENDATIONS

- **People who eat red meat should consume no more than about three portions per week. This is equivalent to about 350–500g (12–18oz) cooked weight of red meat.**

- **Consume very little, if any, processed meat.**

There is strong evidence that consumption of red meat and consumption of processed meat are both causes of colorectal cancer. The recommendation is not to completely avoid eating meat. Meat can be a valuable source of nutrients, in particular protein, iron, zinc and vitamin B_{12}.

> *'For people who eat meat, eat no more than moderate amounts of red meat, such as beef, pork and lamb, and eat little, if any, processed meat.'*
>
> *Opinion of the WCRF Expert panel 2018.*

What is red meat ?

Red meat is any meat that is a dark red colour before being cooked, like beef, pork or lamb. Examples include minced beef, pork chops and roast lamb. There is strong evidence that eating too much red meat can cause bowel cancer, one of the most common cancers in Ireland.

What is processed meat?

Processed meat is meat that is not sold fresh but has been preserved by smoking, curing or salting, or by the addition of preservatives. Examples include ham, bacon, rashers, salami, pepperoni, chorizo, corned beef, as well as hot dogs and sausages.

There is strong evidence that eating too much processed meat can cause bowel and stomach cancer, and may cause pancreatic cancer. Processed meat has actually been classified as a Group 1 carcinogen, or a 'definite' cause of cancer, putting it into the same category as smoking and alcohol. It is more strongly linked to bowel cancer than red meat is.

Both red and processed meats are different from white meats, like chicken or turkey, and from fish, neither of which appear to increase your risk of cancer.

How do red and processed meats cause cancer?

Evidence from large population studies has shown time and time again that people who eat vegetarian diets are at a lower risk for certain cancers. However, it's difficult to say how much of this relates to the absence of meat in their diet, and how much relates to other aspects of their lifestyle, like not smoking, drinking less alcohol, and so on.

We do know that when meat is preserved by smoking, curing or salting, or by the addition of preservatives, cancer-causing substances (carcinogens) can be formed. These substances can damage cells in the body, leading to the development of cancer. Cooking meat at high temperatures, by grilling or barbecuing for example, can also create chemicals in the meat that may increase the risk of cancer. These chemicals are generally produced in higher levels in red and processed meats compared to other meats. It is also believed that the compound that gives red meat its colour, haem, may damage the lining of the bowel, increasing the risk of bowel cancer over time.

Is red meat not good for us?

Red meat is actually a very nourishing and healthy food when consumed in modest amounts. It is an excellent source of nutrients like protein, iron, zinc and vitamin B_{12}. It's certainly not a problem to include small amounts of red meat as part of a healthy, balanced diet. The same cannot be said for processed meats, which have far less nutritional value. If you are a meat-eater, then when choosing meats, it's best to go for the fresh, unprocessed variety.

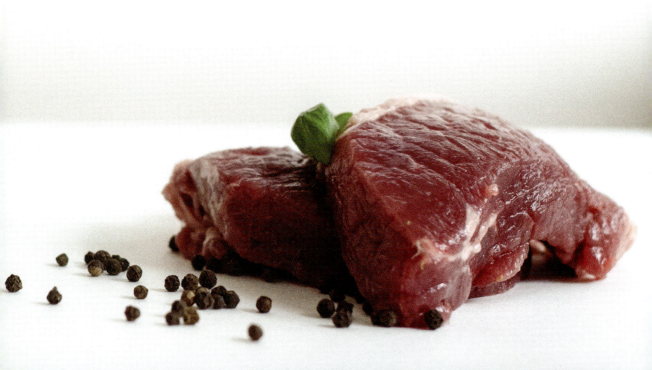

How much is too much?

While the recommendation is to avoid processed meats completely, there is no suggestion that we should switch to a meat-free diet completely, or to a diet containing no foods of animal origin (a vegan diet). Instead, the recommendation states that we should limit our intake of red meat to less than 500g cooked meat (or 750g raw meat) per week. To put this into context, a medium steak weighs about 145g (cooked weight).

For many of us, red meat may be the centrepiece of our main meal several times per week, and this is probably too much. It's really just about being sensible, and not eating too much, too often. Overall, the cancer risks from eating red and processed meats are lower than they are for other things linked to cancer, such as smoking.

How can we cut back on red and processed meats?

There are lots of ways to cut back on red and processed meats without feeling that you're missing out.

- Bulk up with beans. Use kidney beans, chickpeas or lentils to replace some of the meat in dishes such as chilli or bolognese.
- If you're a regular consumer of bacon, chorizo or salami, try spicy chicken or vegetarian sausages instead.
- Eat smaller portions of red meat, and keep a few days in the week red-meat free.
- Choose fish instead – it's delicious, healthy and makes a great alternative to red meat. Sometimes people stick to the battered and breaded varieties, as they aren't sure what to do with fish. Hopefully the fish recipes in this cookbook will give you some great ideas for healthy fish dishes that everyone will love.

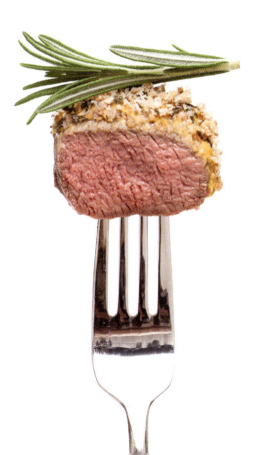

Recommendation 6

Limit consumption of sugar-sweetened drinks.

There is convincing evidence that consumption of sugar-sweetened drinks is a cause of weight gain, overweight and obesity in both children and adults, especially when consumed frequently and in large portions. Sugar-sweetened drinks do this by promoting excess energy (calorie) intake relative to the energy we expend. As outlined already there is strong scientific evidence that greater body fatness is a cause of 12 different cancers.

What is considered a 'sugary drink'?

Sugary drinks refer to drinks with added sugar. They include soda, minerals, sports and energy drinks, barley water, cordial and coffee-and tea-based beverages that have sugars or syrups added to them. They do not include versions of these drinks which are labelled as 'sugar free' or those with artificial sweeteners added. As a lot of sugar is 'hidden' within foods we buy, it is easy to underestimate the amount of sugar we are taking in over the day. It is recommended for an adult with a healthy body weight no more than 30g of added or free sugars should be eaten per day. One teaspoon is proportionate to approximately 5g of sugar, so the recommendation is no more than 6 teaspoons per day. To put this into context, current figures suggest adults are consuming 59g of sugar per day. Most of the sugar we eat comes from food and drink such as soft drinks, cakes, biscuits, sugar, jam, milk products and alcohol. Sugar-sweetened drinks take up a quarter of our daily sugar intake.

In recent years, consumption of sugar-sweetened drinks has increased dramatically, particularly in low- and middle-income countries. While the sale of these drinks has decreased in high-income countries, average daily intakes have remained high. Sugar-sweetened drinks are often consumed with other high-calorie foods. This can lead to greater body fatness.

How does consumption of sweetened drinks affect cancer risk?

Drinking sugary drinks regularly results in overconsumption of calories and leads to weight gain. This excess weight has been associated with an increased risk of 12 different cancers including: mouth, pharynx and larynx, oesophagus (adenocarcinoma), stomach (cardia), pancreas, gallbladder, liver, colon and rectum, breast (postmenopausal), ovary, endometrium, prostate (advanced) and kidney.

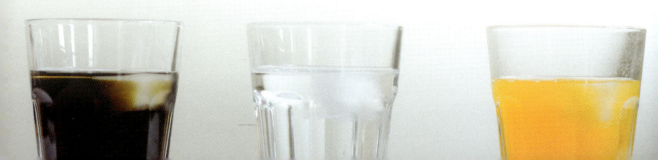

What can I do to reduce my sugar-sweetened drink intake?

Many of the cancer prevention recommendations made by the WCRF tie in together and this recommendation is no different. By increasing the amount of plant foods being eaten (recommendation 4) and reducing the amount of animal foods (recommendation 5) and energy-dense, processed foods (recommendation 3) being consumed, the amount of sugar being consumed will naturally decrease. There are several other ways you can consciously reduce your daily sugar-sweetened drink intake:

- Check food labels. When trying to judge whether drinks are high in a certain nutrient or when comparing drinks, always look at the 'per 100g of food' column. By law, foods must display the nutritional information per 100g of the food for each of the main nutritional components, including sugar. Once you have identified how much sugar is in 100g of the drink, you can use the cut-offs shown in the table below to decide whether the food is high, medium or low in sugar. Use this to choose drinks that are mostly low in sugar and to avoid drinks high in sugar.

AMOUNT OF SUGAR IN 100G OF FOOD		
HIGH	MEDIUM	LOW
Over 15g	5g to 15g	Less than 5g

- Choose 'no added sugar' or 'low sugar' varieties. As sugar has been well-documented as an unhealthy additive to food, many manufacturers have taken note and released 'no added sugar' or 'low sugar' varieties of their products. For example, fizzy drinks are usually extremely high in sugar, however many large brands have released low-sugar drinks to give consumers more control over their sugar content.

- To maintain adequate hydration, it is best to drink water or unsweetened drinks such as tea or coffee with no added sugar. Fruit juices are recommended to be consumed in small amounts, as even unsweetened juices can cause weight gain in a similar way to sugar-sweetened drinks. Scientific research has found that artificially sweetened drinks do not play a strong role in overweight/obesity or cancer occurrence.

Recommendation 7

Limit alcohol consumption.

For cancer prevention it's best not to drink alcohol.

Alcohol causes cancer

The International Agency for Research on Cancer (IARC) has classified alcohol as a group 1 carcinogen. This is the risk category and means that there is 'convincing evidence' that alcohol causes cancer in humans. The strongest evidence is in relation to cancers of the mouth, throat, larynx (voice box), oesophagus (squamous cell carcinoma), liver, colorectum (bowel), stomach, and breast (pre- and post-menopause).

There is no safe level of alcohol when it comes to cancer. Simply put, the risk of alcohol-related cancers increases the more you drink. And the less alcohol you drink, the lower your risk of these cancers. Drinking no alcohol at all offers the best possible protection against alcohol-related cancers. The cancer risks from alcohol are the same regardless of the type of alcoholic beverage consumed (wine, beer, spirits, etc). It is the ethanol, or pure alcohol, rather than any other ingredient of the alcoholic beverage that causes cancer.

How does alcohol increase the risk of cancer?

Alcohol increases the risk of cancer in a number of different ways. Firstly alcohol is a carcinogen. It is converted in our bodies to a toxic chemical called acetaldehyde. This can cause cancer by damaging our DNA and stopping cells from repairing the damage. Alcohol can also increase the levels of some hormones, such as oestrogen, which particularly increases the risk of breast cancer.

Is alcohol-related cancer a problem in Ireland?

Yes, more than you might imagine. According to the National Cancer Control Programme, 900 people are diagnosed with alcohol-related cancers every year in Ireland, and some 500 people will die from these diseases. Alcohol is responsible for 1 in 8 breast cancers in Ireland. The proportion of alcohol-related deaths from cancer in Ireland is higher than the European average, and rates in Europe are the highest globally.

In Irish men, the majority of alcohol-related cancer deaths occur due to cancers of the mouth, throat and larynx. The risk of developing these cancers is far greater in those who smoke and drink, compared to those who do one or the other.

In women, most alcohol-related cancer deaths occur due to breast cancer. Irish women are now drinking more alcohol, more often, than previous generations, and it is having very real cancer implications. Consuming just one standard drink per day (e.g. one small glass of wine) is associated with a 9% increase in the risk of developing breast cancer, compared to non-drinkers. Consuming 3 to 6 standard drinks per day increases the risk of breast cancer by 41%, compared to a non-drinker. A full bottle of wine at 12.5% alcohol contains about 7 standard drinks, meaning the risk of developing breast cancer is significantly increased in women who consume the equivalent of a half bottle of wine, or more, daily.

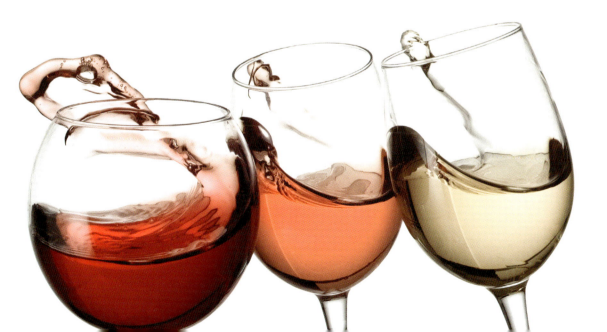

But I thought drinking in moderation was supposed to be good for me?

There is evidence that modest amounts of alcohol may reduce the risk of coronary heart disease in people who are already at some risk (e.g. in older adults with high cholesterol). For these people, there is a recommendation to take modest amounts of alcohol daily where there is no risk of addiction (although the benefits are not considered strong enough to encourage non-drinkers to take up alcohol). This is not the case for cancer. Because of the strong scientific evidence that drinking all types of alcoholic drinks can increase your risk of cancer, it is recommended that individuals do not drink alcohol at all.

What can we do to reduce our cancer risk?

Ideally in terms of cancer prevention zero alcohol consumption is best. However, for those that choose to drink, staying within the low-risk weekly guidelines for alcohol consumption could prevent over half of all alcohol-related cancers in Ireland. The guidelines are:

- For men, no more than 17 standard drinks spread out over the course of a week, with at least 2–3 alcohol-free days
- For women, no more than 11 standard drinks spread out over the course of a week, with at least 2–3 alcohol-free days

In Ireland, one standard drink contains around 10g of ethanol, or pure alcohol. Here are some examples of one standard drink:

- A pub measure of spirits (35.5ml)

- A small glass of wine (100ml)

- A half pint of normal-strength beer

- An alcopop (275ml bottle)

For those individuals drinking more than this at present, aiming to meet these guidelines would be a great start. In terms of cancer risk, however, it would be better still to reduce our alcohol consumption to levels below this.

Alcohol has long been a part of Irish culture. We use it to celebrate, to relax and to commiserate. A shift in this culture is unlikely, but it's important that we are aware of the extent of the alcohol and cancer relationship. Then, at least, we have the choice to reduce our intake and give ourselves a better outlook in terms of cancer risk. So, why not offer to be the designated driver on a night out? Or try a lower-strength beer or wine? Or a tasty spritzer or shandy? Your body will thank you in the long term for it.

Recommendation 8

Do not use supplements for cancer prevention.

Aim to meet nutritional needs through diet alone.

What are dietary supplements?

Dietary supplements are generally a blend of vitamins, minerals, herbs/plant material. They can be taken in pill, capsule, tablet or liquid form. On the island of Ireland, one in four of us are taking dietary supplements at any given time, often to make up for what we feel is a lack in our normal diet.

'For most people consumption of the right food and drink is more likely to protect against cancer than dietary supplements.'

WCRF Expert report 2018

Can dietary supplements reduce our risk of cancer?

It can be difficult to find reliable information about dietary supplements and their usefulness in preventing cancer, as media reports tend to exaggerate claims about supplements and health. Supplements are also marketed in a way that can make you believe they are capable of dramatically improving your health and wellbeing.

Our best available evidence shows that while certain high-dose dietary supplements may be protective against cancer, others can actually increase your cancer risk. However, the studies that showed these effects were all carried out on very specific groups of people – like smokers, people exposed to asbestos and those with known nutrient deficiencies – so they may not be relevant to the general public.

The World Cancer Research Fund recommends that dietary supplements are not taken for the purpose of cancer prevention. Instead, they recommend that we meet nutritional needs through diet alone. For most people, eating a healthy, balanced diet will give a better chance of protecting against cancers than any supplement ever could.

Does anyone really need to take supplements?

While taking supplements cannot fully correct a poor diet, they can be very useful where somebody is ill or has a poor diet. For instance, frail older people with a poor food intake might benefit from a regular, low-dose multivitamin and mineral supplement. In Ireland, all women who could become pregnant are recommended to take a 400µg folic acid supplement daily, to protect against the risk of neural tube defects in babies. In addition, during pregnancy many women are advised by their doctors to take an iron supplement. Likewise, it is recommended that babies in Ireland are given a 5µg vitamin D supplement daily from birth to twelve months to protect against vitamin D deficiency in this group.

What about people going through cancer treatment?

Dietary supplements are widely used by people with cancer to help fight their cancer or make them feel better.

While most supplements are safe for people to use alongside conventional cancer treatments, there is a risk that some types of supplements could interact with particular types of cancer drugs. For this reason, it's really important for cancer patients to get advice from their doctor before starting to take any dietary supplement.

During the course of cancer treatment, your doctor may prescribe dietary supplements in certain situations. For example, if your treatment involves hormonal therapy that could weaken your bones, your doctor may prescribe calcium and vitamin D supplements. Or if you are finding it difficult to eat a normal, balanced diet due to the cancer or its treatment, your doctor may recommend a good-quality, daily multivitamin and mineral supplement, to be taken at the stated dose.

What should we take instead of dietary supplements to prevent cancer?

In a nutshell – good food! At the moment, we have no reliable evidence that any type of dietary supplement can help to prevent cancer in most people. But we do know that a healthy diet with plenty of fruit and vegetables can reduce cancer risk for everybody. Without a doubt, the best source of nourishment is food. Foods and drinks contain a whole host of potentially beneficial constituents that we simply cannot get from supplements alone. They also give us natural combinations of nutrients that work together to keep us healthy, something that supplements cannot achieve as well.

A healthy, balanced diet that follows the recommendations within this book will give a far better chance of avoiding cancer than any individual dietary supplement can.

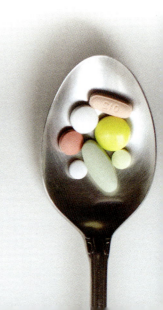

Recommendation 9

For mothers: breastfeed your baby, if you can.

Breastfeeding is good for both mother and baby.

PERSONAL RECOMMENDATIONS

- Aim to breastfeed infants exclusively up to 6 months and then up to 2 years or beyond alongside appropriate complementary feeding.

There is 'strong' evidence that breastfeeding decreases the risk of breast cancer in the mother (WCRF Expert Report 2018).

This recommendation has two separate parts to it: mothers to breastfeed, and children to be breastfed. The wording is intentional, and refers to the cancer prevention benefits that exist for both mother and child where a baby is breastfed. The World Cancer Research Fund recommends that babies be 'exclusively breastfed' for the first 6 months of life, meaning that babies should take nothing other than breast milk during this time (no solid foods, infant formula or water). They also recommend 'sustained breastfeeding' or feeding that continues until the baby is at least 2 years old, with suitable weaning foods introduced around the age of 6 months.

Sustained, exclusive breastfeeding has historically been the norm. It is only in relatively recent times that this has changed, with the development and marketing of infant formulas, initially in high-income countries. Ireland has long held one of the lowest rates of breastfeeding in the world, but thankfully, recent years have seen a slow but steady rise in the number of Irish mothers choosing to breastfeed. Many of the benefits of breastfeeding are well established. Breast milk contains all the nutrients a baby needs – in the perfect quantities – for healthy growth and development. It also contains antibodies which help the baby build a strong immune system, meaning there is less chance they will suffer diarrhoea, constipation or chest and ear infections. Breastfed babies are less likely to develop the atopic conditions: allergies, asthma and eczema. Breastfeeding becomes particularly vital in parts of the world where water supplies are not safe and families may not readily have the money to buy infant formula. What may be less well known, however, is that breastfeeding also plays a role in protecting both mother and baby against certain cancers into the future.

How does breastfeeding protect babies against cancers?

Breastfeeding helps babies to grow at a healthy rate. Babies who are breastfed are less likely to become overweight or obese as children compared to babies fed on infant formula. And the longer a baby is breastfed, the lower their risk of becoming overweight or obese. There are a number of theories as to why this happens. One widely held view is that breastfed babies learn to control the amount of human milk and calories they consume better than bottle-fed babies, who are often encouraged to finish a bottle after they are satisfied. Since a child's weight usually tracks into adulthood, babies who are breastfed are also less likely to become overweight or obese as adults.

This is really important, because being a healthy weight as an adult reduces our risk of developing 12 different cancers – including breast and bowel cancers – as well as other diseases like heart disease and Type 2 diabetes. In fact, staying at a healthy weight is one of the most important things we can do to reduce our cancer risk (see recommendation 1, page 10).

How does breastfeeding protect mothers against cancer?

There is strong evidence that mothers who breastfeed are at a reduced risk for breast cancer for the rest of their lives. And the longer a mother breastfeeds for, the stronger that protection is. As well as helping babies to gain weight steadily, breastfeeding helps new mothers to lose the baby weight steadily and regain their pre-pregnancy figures. During pregnancy, a woman's body stores around seven pounds of fat specifically for the purpose of nourishing her baby after birth, so the subsequent loss of this fat store through the production of breast milk is ideal. This weight loss alone can help reduce a woman's risk of breast cancer, as breast cancer is strongly related to weight. But breastfeeding also temporarily lowers levels of oestrogen and other hormones in the mother's body, which helps to reduce her risk of breast cancer. And remarkably, at the end of breastfeeding, a woman's body gets rid of any cells in the breasts that may have DNA damage, further reducing the chances of breast cancer developing in the future. There is some evidence to suggest that breastfeeding may protect women against ovarian cancer, but this evidence is more limited.

A final word

While the WCRF recommends that infants be exclusively breastfed for the first 6 months of life, only a small proportion of mothers currently meet this recommendation (18% in Europe and 1% in Ireland), although the practice is increasing. It's worth remembering that any time spent breastfeeding provides some benefit for mother and baby, but that the longer breastfeeding continues, the greater the health protection for both.

Despite its many health benefits, breastfeeding isn't easy. Anybody who has tried it, or supported a new mother in the early days of breastfeeding, will appreciate that it is a skill that both mother and baby must learn. Good support from partners, family members and healthcare professionals is essential to making things work – so we can all play a part in helping to make this recommendation a reality, and giving the next generation of Irish babies the best possible start in life.

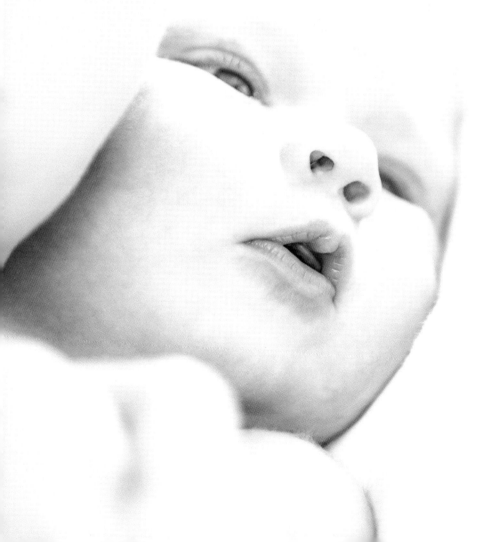

After a cancer diagnosis

After a cancer diagnosis: follow the WCRF recommendations, if you can. Check with your health professional what is right for you.

PERSONAL RECOMMENDATIONS

- All cancer survivors to receive nutritional care from an appropriately trained professional.
- Unless otherwise advised, and if they can, all cancer survivors are advised to follow the cancer prevention recommendations as far as possible after the acute stage of treatment.

The term 'cancer survivor' describes anyone who has been given a diagnosis of cancer at any stage, including those who have recovered from the disease.

When it comes to taking responsibility for their health, cancer survivors are a motivated group. They tend to be very receptive to advice from their medical and surgical teams. So what should people living with cancer do? Are the circumstances of people who have recovered from cancer any different from those of people free from cancer? When it comes to family shopping and meal preparation, should the person with cancer be treated differently? Or should the whole family follow the same recommendations and advice?

Ultimately, research into how to prevent cancers recurring is in its early days. The World Cancer Research Fund (WCRF) has pledged that research into how best to improve the health of cancer survivors will take priority in the scientific work it funds into the future. For now, however, it has examined all available evidence to come up with the following recommendation:

If able to do so, and unless otherwise advised, cancer survivors should aim to follow the WCRF recommendations for diet, healthy weight and physical activity.

The evidence shows that eating a mainly plant-based diet, staying at a healthy weight and keeping physically active will help lower the chances of cancers recurring. Following these recommendations will also improve the chances of longer-term survival after a cancer, particularly breast cancer.

It is also recommended that cancer survivors receive nutritional care from an appropriately qualified professional, like a registered dietitian. There is an abundance of information out there on diet for cancer survivors, but unfortunately it comes from many different sources and is often conflicting or incorrect. A healthcare professional who can evaluate the scientific evidence around a specific diet or dietary supplement, and then advise the cancer survivor based on their own unique medical situation, would be ideal.

Should all cancer survivors follow these recommendations?

Not quite – there are exceptions. These recommendations do not apply to anybody going through cancer treatments at present. If you have recently been diagnosed with cancer, or are currently undergoing treatment for cancer, your nutritional needs are likely to be unique right now. In this case, it is more important to follow your doctor's advice. You may be referred to the book *Good Nutrition for Cancer Recovery* (which is a free resource available in your local hospital or from www.breakthroughcancerresearch.ie), which contains recipes with a higher protein and calorie content, suitable for most people with a new diagnosis of cancer.

If you are a cancer survivor whose treatments have affected your ability to eat or digest certain foods, then you may also have specific dietary requirements to consider. Patients who have undergone removal of part of the stomach (gastrectomy) or colon (colectomy), for example, may have particular digestive issues that call for a more specialised type of diet. A registered dietitian with experience in oncology would be ideally placed to advise on this.

Nothing to lose ...

While there can never be a guarantee against cancer returning, the best evidence we have at the moment is simply to try and follow the recommendations by the World Cancer Research Fund which are discussed within this book. The good news is that aiming for a healthy weight, staying physically active and eating a mainly plant-based diet is likely to reduce our risk of other chronic diseases – like heart disease or Type 2 diabetes – as well as cancer. And regular physical activity is one of the most effective ways we have of relieving stress, reducing anxiety and bringing a sense of control over our circumstances. So, in following this recommendation, there really is nothing to lose, and only good things to gain.

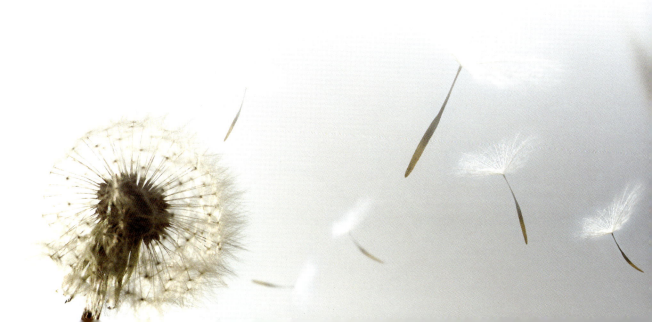

Common myths and misconceptions

Below we discuss some of the most common myths and misconceptions that exist in relation to diet and cancer prevention. It is important to say that many myths are routed in science but the degree of truth or the extent to which they apply to the general population can vary greatly. Science is constantly evolving, so new evidence and information is always coming to the fore. That means that advice and information will change over time, but until there is evidence proving or disproving something, it would be unsafe to advise it or advise against it. In general, a balanced diet rich in fruit, vegetables, wholegrains and pulses, with limited amounts of animal products, is the key to optimising your health through eating.

Does sugar feed cancer?

Although science has shown that cancer cells consume sugar (glucose), no human studies have shown that eating sugar will fuel cancer growth, or that avoiding sugar will halt the growth of cancer cells.

Focusing on the fact that cancer cells consume sugar is an oversimplification of a complex process. When we eat sugar, sugary foods or any carbohydrate (fruit, vegetables, bread, pasta, rice, cereals, potatoes, yogurt, etc), they are broken down or converted to glucose in our body. Simple sugars (e.g. table sugar) are broken down into glucose a lot quicker than complex carbohydrates (e.g. porridge). Every single cell within our body then uses glucose to survive and perform its duty. If we don't consume carbohydrate, our body will convert fat and protein into glucose as a last resort because we need a supply of glucose in order to keep our cells alive. There's no way to provide our body's cells with the glucose they critically need, and still 'starve' cancer cells of glucose. In addition, cancer cells need other nutrients to survive, they don't run solely on glucose (or sugar).

We do know there is an indirect link between sugar and cancer. Consuming excess sugar will promote weight gain and this weight gain will increase your risk of developing cancer. For this reason, it is important to limit intakes of refined sugars, added sugars and energy-dense foods. This is discussed in more detail in recommendation 6, page 26.

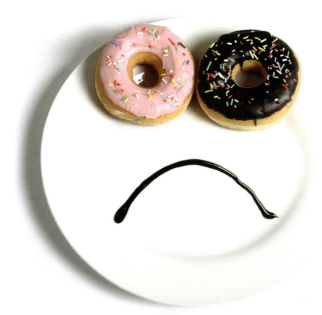

Do artificial sweeteners cause cancer?

No. Extensive studies have been performed to investigate the safety of artificial sweeteners. No evidence was found to link the use of artificial sweeteners and the development of cancer. Furthermore, as is the case for all food additives, sweeteners are regulated by the European Food Safety Authority (EFSA). This means that they undergo rigorous safety testing and risk assessment before being allowed to go on the market in Europe. They will only be allowed go on sale if they have been deemed safe to use by EFSA and EFSA will continually review the scientific evidence and re-evaluate their decisions. Research has shown that artificial sweeteners are safe to consume up to a certain level (the Acceptable Daily Intake (ADI)) in the general population. This excludes infants and young children as the use of artificial sweeteners is not recommended in these groups. The ADI is different for each type of artificial sweetener but people would have to be using an excessive amount of sweetener to reach this level. Moderate use is completely safe.

(For example, ADI for aspartame is 40mg/kg body weight/per day (for a 70kg individual this means 2800mg/day) and there is an average of 180mg of aspartame in a can of Diet Coke.)

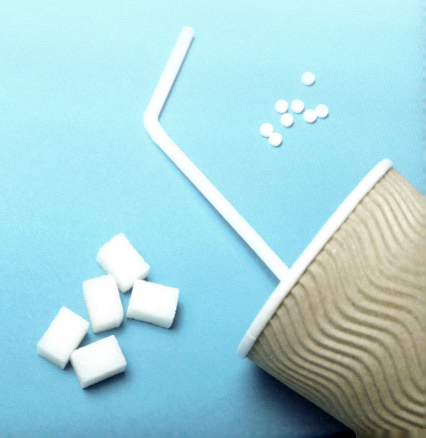

Do dairy products cause cancer?

There is no strong evidence to suggest a link between dairy products and increased cancer risk. There is strong evidence that dairy products reduce the risk of colorectal cancer (WCRF 2017) and 'limited evidence' that dairy products decrease the risk of pre-menopausal breast cancer and that diets high in calcium can decrease the risk of both pre- and post-menopausal breast cancer. The myth that dairy is linked with cancer often comes from concerns the public have surrounding the addition of hormones to milk and meat products. In Europe, the addition of hormones to milk or meat is strictly banned and the sale of meat from countries where the addition of hormones is allowed is also illegal. As a result, concerns over the presence of these hormones in dairy or meat products in Europe are unfounded.

Is organic food better?

Organic foods are those grown without using artificial fertilisers, pesticides or chemicals. Organic foods are generally more expensive and are becoming increasingly popular due to claims that the produce is safer and more nutritious. However, the nutritional composition of foods is not altered when grown organically so organic fruit and vegetables have the same nutritional composition as non-organic varieties. On top of this, there is no strong evidence to link organic foods with a reduced risk of cancer. In Europe, the level of pesticides on food is tightly regulated and food safety authorities have a responsibility to ensure the levels in foods are well within safe limits. Fruit and vegetables are key components of a cancer-prevention diet so the main priority is to include them however you can: organic, non-organic, fresh, frozen, tinned – they all count!

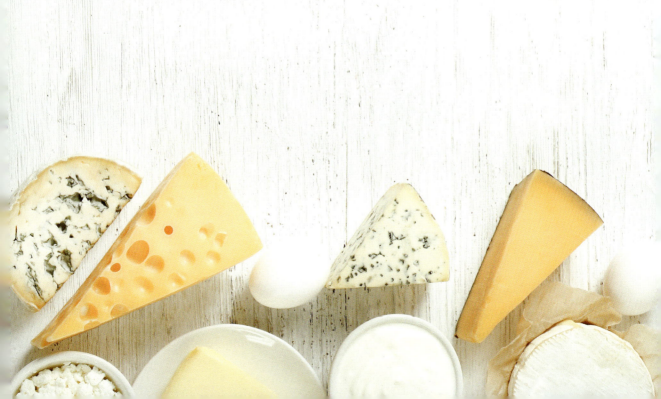

Can superfoods protect against cancer?

'Superfoods' are foods that are claimed to possess potent nutritional benefits that enhance health and protect against diseases such as cancer. Acai berries, blueberries, chia seeds, kale, garlic, turmeric... the list of foods promoted as having 'superfood' properties is endless.

Claims surrounding superfoods are often very misleading as they are usually based on results of studies looking at the effect of nutrients on cells in the lab. Although these studies give us important results, the findings cannot be automatically translated to human diets, for a number of reasons. Firstly, we don't eat nutrients, we eat whole foods. A nutrient in isolation may cause a different response than if consumed within a whole food. Secondly, the nutrients being investigated are often studied at very high levels, levels much higher than what we would be able to eat in our diet. Finally, our bodies also don't act the same way cells do in laboratory studies. The relationships seen at cellular level might not exist at a whole body level. So we need large-scale population studies before we can make recommendations on individual nutrients.

In reality, there is no such thing as a superfood. No single food has the ability to 'undo' the effect of an unhealthy diet or lifestyle. Foods that have demonstrated beneficial properties are best incorporated as part of a healthy diet, along with a wide variety of other healthy foods. Instead of focusing on 'superfoods', we should focus on 'superdiets'. A 'superdiet' for cancer prevention is a balanced diet that is rich in a variety of fruit, vegetables, wholegrains and pulses, with limited amounts of animal products.

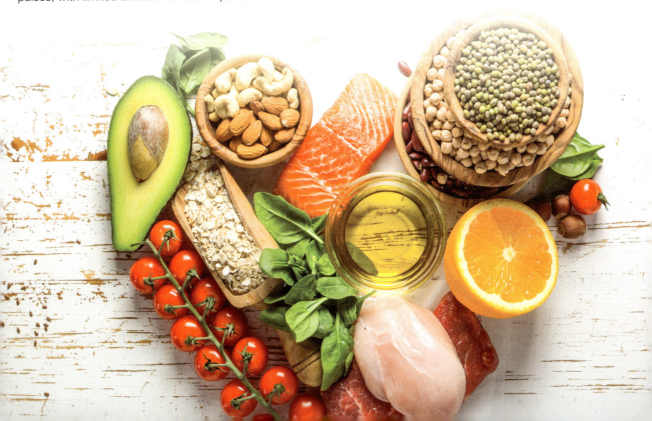

Store cupboard essentials

We all live busy lives and it can be really challenging to try to eat healthily when you are short on time. A well-stocked cupboard will help you to create nutritious meals when you are in a hurry. Tinned, dried and frozen foods are time-saving nutritious essentials that you can stock up on and store until needed. A selection of herbs and spices is particularly important for flavouring your food without adding salt, and having a variety of tinned beans in the cupboard will allow you to whip up protein-rich meat-less meals. We have compiled a list of foods below, the majority of which are non-perishable, which will help you to create a well-rounded food pantry. Although your first 'stock-up' shop may be expensive, you will then have the ingredients on hand for when you need them. The ingredients can be mixed and matched or else paired with frozen foods (see page 43) or a few key fresh ingredients to make a variety of delicious, healthy meals.

Tins

- Tinned tomatoes – chopped tomatoes, plum tomatoes, passata
- Sweetcorn
- Tinned beans – kidney beans, mixed beans, butter beans
- Baked beans (opt for reduced sugar and salt varieties)
- Chickpeas
- Tinned fish – tuna, salmon, mackerel, sardines (opt for varieties tinned in spring water or tomato sauce)
- Light coconut milk
- Tinned pineapple (in natural juice)

Pulses and grains

- Wholegrain rice
- Brown pasta
- Brown noodles
- Quinoa
- Lentils

Other

- Nuts and seeds
- Dried fruit
- Oats
- Flour – brown, white and cornflour

Herbs and spices

- Cumin (ground, seeds)
- Coriander (ground, seeds)
- Smoked paprika
- Chilli (powder, flakes)
- Turmeric
- Cayenne
- Cardamom seeds
- Fennel seeds
- Mustard seeds

Condiments, sauces and jars

- Fats – olive oil, vegetable oil, low-calorie spray
- Black pepper
- Low salt/sodium stock cubes
- Tomato puree
- Tomato ketchup (opt for reduced sugar and salt varieties)
- Light mayonnaise
- Mustard – wholegrain, Dijon
- Horseradish sauce
- Worcestershire sauce
- Low salt/sodium soy sauce
- Vinegars – red wine, balsamic, apple cider vinegar
- Olives
- Sundried tomato paste
- Vanilla extract
- Honey
- Nut butter

Key fresh products

- Lean meats
- Fish
- Eggs
- Vegetables of choice
- Fruit of choice
- Fresh herbs
- Low-fat milk, low-fat natural yogurt, low-fat crème fraiche, low-fat cheese

Making use of your freezer

Your freezer is an important asset in your kitchen and can be used along with your store cupboard to create a selection of convenient, nutritionally balanced meals. The key to making the most of your freezer is organisation. Freezer space can be an issue, so freezing foods in freezer bags instead of containers will free up a lot of space. It is important to label and date everything so you can keep track of what needs to be used up and when. As a rule of thumb, foods should not be stored in a freezer for longer than 6 months and only freezers that run at -18°C are suitable for long-term freezing (3–6 months).

Foods should be frozen when as fresh as possible and if you are freezing cooked food it needs to have cooled to at least room temperature before being put in the freezer. Foods can only be defrosted once and should always be defrosted in a fridge rather than at room temperature. Only defrost food in a microwave if you are cooking it immediately after defrosting. Foods can only be re-frozen if they have been cooked to piping hot (>70°C) and you can only perform this step once (Food Safety Authority of Ireland (FSAI)). Be mindful of portion sizes when you are freezing foods. If you freeze a batch of food together you will have to defrost the entire batch, which could result in wastage. Freezing foods in individual portions will allow you to only defrost the amount that you need.

Most foods are suitable for freezing and it is a great way of taking the hassle out of meal preparation, as well as preventing food waste. Chopping ingredients like garlic, chilli or ginger can be tedious and in general you won't be using up an entire bulb of garlic or root of ginger in one go. When you are preparing something like garlic for a meal, chop extra and freeze it in an ice-cube tray in a small amount of water. Then when you are short on time or don't have fresh garlic in the house you can pop the frozen garlic out of the tray and into your pot/pan. This is also a really handy way of storing lemon and lime juice or fresh herbs that tend to off quite quickly. If you have lots of vegetables lying around, you can prepare them and freeze vegetable mixes in freezer bags for days when you don't have time to chop everything up.

You can also use the freezer to get the most out of leftover bread. You can freeze slices of bread or blitz the remainder of a loaf in a food processer to make breadcrumbs. You will see any recipes in this cookbook that use breadcrumbs recommend crumbs made from wholemeal bread (as it is higher in fibre). The next time you have wholemeal bread left over, blitz it to make breadcrumbs and freeze it. Then when you have a recipe that calls for wholemeal breadcrumbs you can take a handful from your store. Breadcrumbs defrost very quickly and can be used from frozen, so they are really handy to have in the freezer.

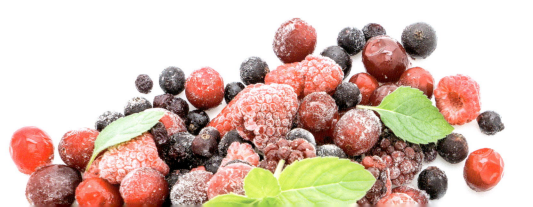

Below is a list of some of the most useful things to keep stocked in your freezer.

- Chopped garlic
- Chopped chilli
- Chopped/grated ginger
- Chopped onion
- Chopped prepared vegetable mixes
- Frozen vegetables, e.g. frozen peas, corn on the cob

- Frozen mixed berries
- Lemon and lime juice frozen in ice-cube trays/bags
- Wholemeal breadcrumbs
- Bread
- Frozen meat/fish/prawns
- Leftovers

Top tips for cooking healthily

- Keep your store cupboard well stocked.
- Make use of your freezer.
- Aim to have a vegetarian dinner at least 2 days a week.
- Choose non-meat sources of protein at lunchtime, e.g. fish, eggs, beans, pulses.
- Choose lean cuts of meat.
- Choose healthier cooking methods. Opt for steaming, stir-frying, baking, boiling or grilling instead of frying, deep-frying or roasting in fat.
- Choose low-fat varieties of foods, e.g. low-fat yogurt, low-fat cheese, low-fat mayonnaise.
- Use homemade or low salt/sodium stock cubes to cut down on your salt intake.
- You don't have to stir-fry in fat, you can stir-fry in water in order to cut back on calories. Use a tbsp. of water instead of oil and keep an eye on the pan to make sure that it does not dry out. If it gets dry, just keep adding water, tablespoon by tablespoon. Similarly if you use oil when frying food and the pan gets dry or starts to stick, add water instead of more oil.
- Eat a rainbow – including a wide variety of different coloured fruit and vegetables will help to make sure you are eating a wide range of nutrients.

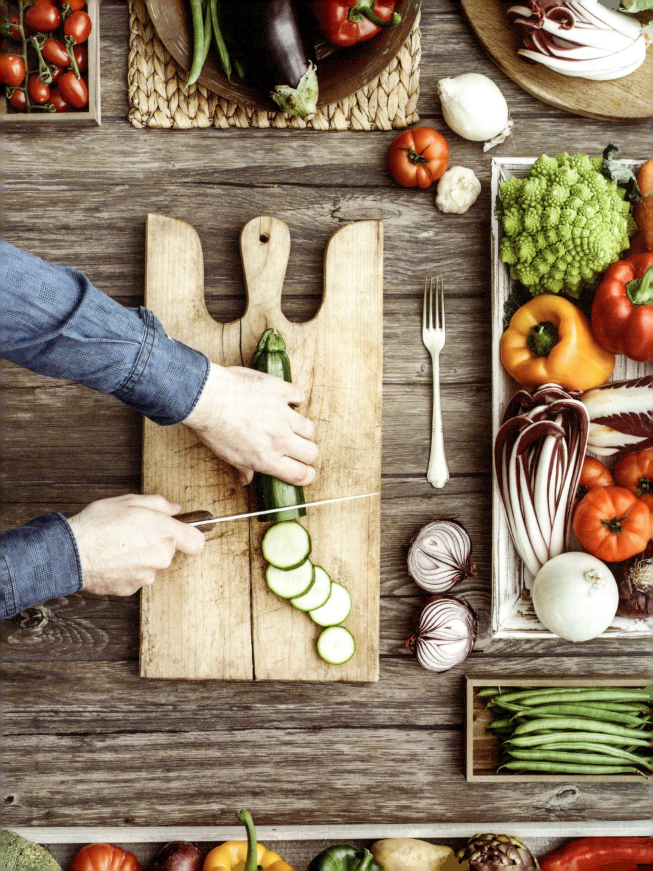

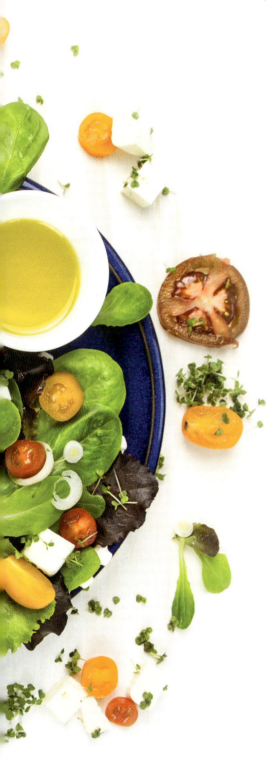

Recipes

LIGHT MEALS

SOUP

Butternut squash soup

Carrot and coriander soup

Chicken and vegetable soup

Lentil and spinach soup

Minestrone

Moroccan roasted vegetable and chickpea soup

Pea and mint soup

Red lentil and tomato soup

Roast chicken soup

Tomato and cannellini bean soup

Tomato and roasted red pepper soup

Vegetable soup

BREAD

Oat bread

Soda bread

Brown bread with seeds

SALADS

Crunchy tossed salad

Chickpea and mango salad

Salmon and pasta salad

Italian salad

Quinoa with roasted vegetables and feta

Three-grain salad

Quick salad with berries

Warm chicken salad with French dressing

Warm shredded chicken and chilli salad

Rainbow salad

Pink tabbouleh salad

Roast squash, bean and kale salad

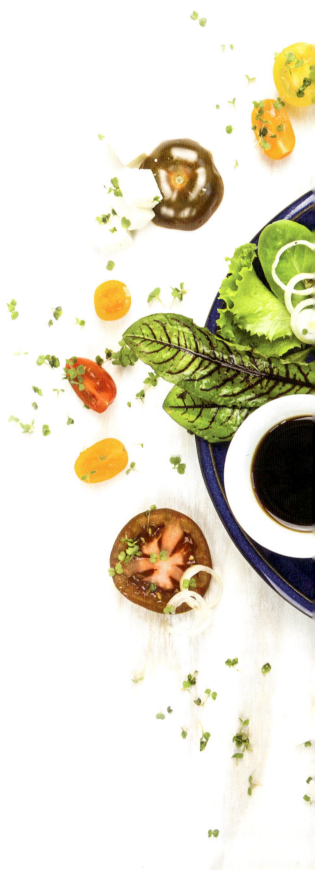

HOT LIGHT MEALS

Chicken fajita stuffed peppers

Courgette and feta fritters

Ranch-style eggs

Spinach and sweet potato tortilla

Mexican beans on toast

Tuna and sweetcorn fritters

Baked potatoes:

- With bean chilli
- With beef chilli
- With chicken, onion and cheese
- With salmon
- With tuna and sweetcorn
- With baked beans

Healthy omelette

Tortilla pizza

Farmers market scramble

SANDWICHES AND WRAPS

Chicken pesto wrap

Spicy chicken pitta

Falafel wraps

Pitta with chicken, carrot and coriander salad

Healthy sandwich fillings

HEALTHY SNACKS AND SAVOURY DIPS

Homemade tortilla chips

Vegetable crudités

Butter bean and almond dip

Easy guacamole

Red pepper hummus

Homemade tzatziki dip

Oil-free hummus

Aubergine and coriander dip

Healthy coleslaw

Spicy mango salsa

Tomato and chilli salsa

White bean dip

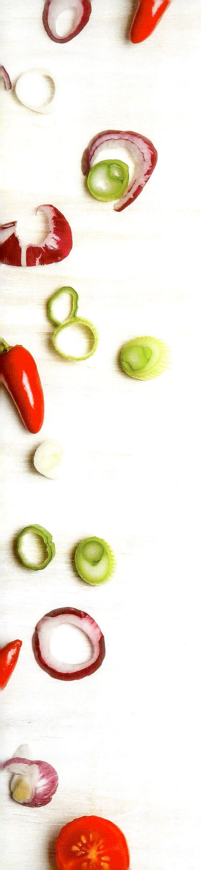

MAIN MEALS

RED MEAT
Beef burgers
Beef stew
Beef stroganoff
Chilli con carne
Italian meatballs with pasta
Lamb tagine
Healthy lasagne
Shepherd's pie
Spaghetti bolognese
Spiced pork tray bake
Steak with salsa verde
Sweet and sour pork

POULTRY
Chicken and broccoli bake
Chicken casserole
Chicken goujons
Chicken, bean and kale stew
Chicken stir-fry with cashew nuts
Fruity chicken tagine
Grilled chicken with green lentil dahl
Tandoori chicken fillet burger
Turkey fajitas
Pasta with turkey, almond and rocket
Chicken Lahori
Creamy chicken and tomato bake
Chicken and mushroom risotto
Spicy sweet Thai noodles with chicken

FISH
Baked cod with a vine tomato topping
Fish pie
Fish cakes
Fisherman's stew
Glazed salmon

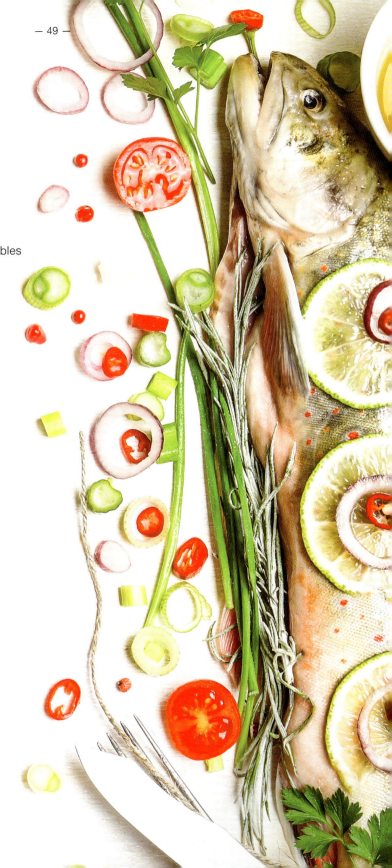

Grilled lemon-scented salmon with chickpea, tomato and spinach ragout

Healthy fish and chips

Mediterranean fish tray bake

Prawn paella

Salmon linguine

Seared haddock with horseradish aioli

Pasta with mackerel and Mediterranean vegetables

Baked hake/cod with a herb crust

Spicy Italian cod

VEGETARIAN

Bean chilli

Butternut squash, chickpea and spinach curry

Pasta arrabbiata

Egg-fried rice

Healthy pizza

Millet, sweet potato and cashew burgers

Kidney bean and potato curry

Ratatouille

Roast tomato and orzo bake

Stuffed mushrooms

Vegetable and red lentil pie

Vegetable jalfrezi

Butter bean stew

Kale, tomato and lemon spaghetti

Vegetarian casserole

Quorn pie

Spicy rice and lentil one-pot

SIDE DISHES

Champ mash potato

Mustard mash

Roast garlic baby potatoes

Spicy potato wedges

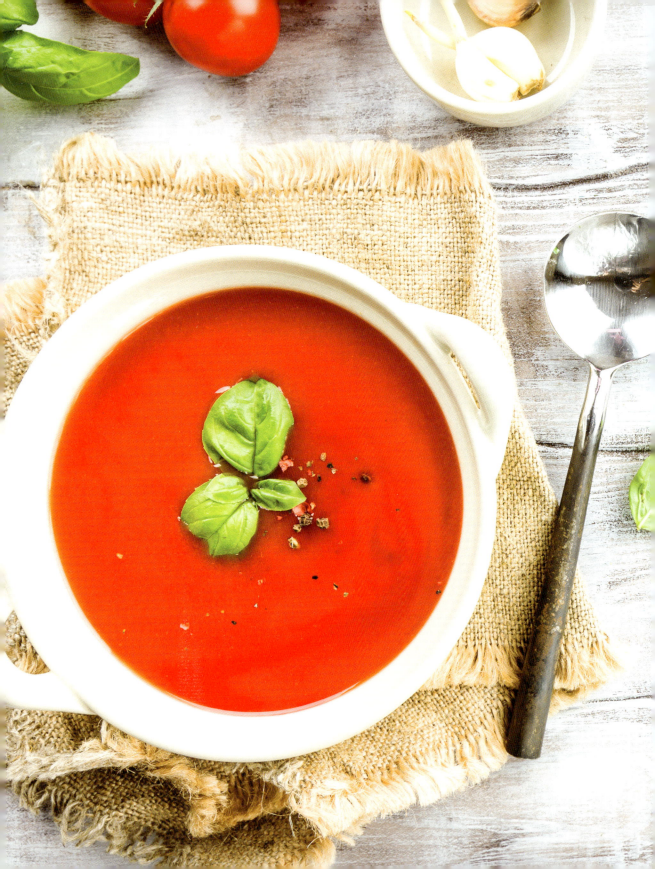

Soup

Butternut squash soup

Carrot and coriander soup

Chicken and vegetable soup

Lentil and spinach soup

Minestrone

Moroccan roasted vegetable and chickpea soup

Pea and mint soup

Red lentil and tomato soup

Roast chicken soup

Tomato and cannellini bean soup

Tomato and roasted red pepper soup

Vegetable soup

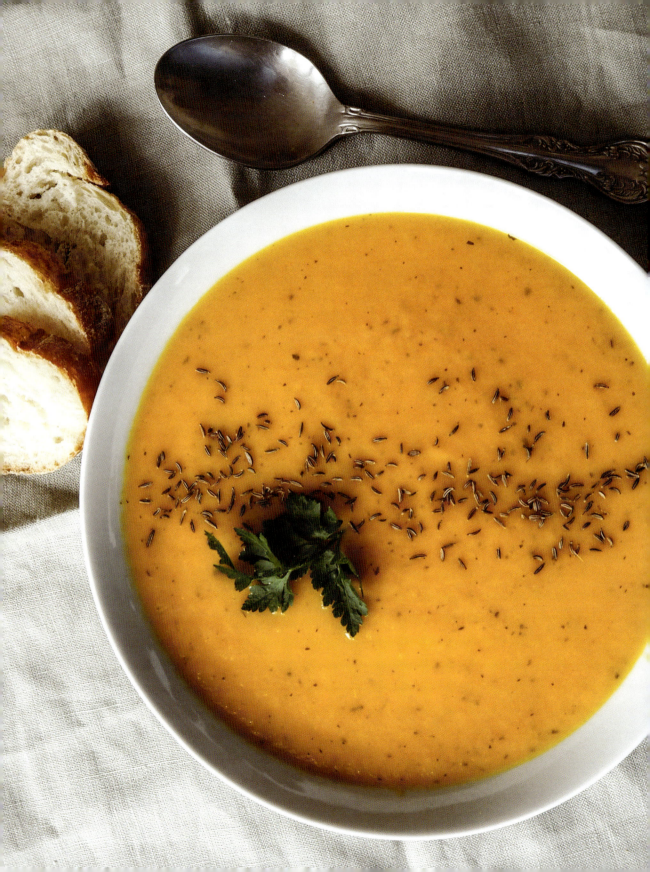

Butternut squash soup

Serves: 5–6 (makes 2l) **Prep time:** 15 mins **Cooking time:** 40 mins

Ingredients

- 2 tbsp. olive oil
- 3 carrots, chopped
- 1 butternut squash, peeled and chopped
- 2 small onions, peeled and finely chopped
- 1 leek, washed and chopped
- 3 sticks celery, finely chopped
- ½ tsp. grated ginger
- ½ tsp. ground cumin
- Freshly ground black pepper
- 1400ml/6 cups stock approximately

Method

1. Heat the oven to 200°C/400°F (fan 180°C/350°F) or gas mark 6 and roast the carrot and squash with 1 tbsp. of the oil for 30 minutes.

2. Meanwhile heat the remaining oil in a large pan and fry the onion, leek and celery for 5 minutes until softened.

3. Add the squash, carrots, ginger, cumin and ground black pepper and fry for another 5 minutes.

4. Add the stock or water and cook on a gentle heat until vegetables are soft, about 10 minutes.

5. Blend with a hand blender.

NUTRITION INFORMATION
Amount per serving

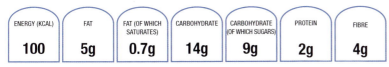

ENERGY (KCAL)	FAT	FAT (OF WHICH SATURATES)	CARBOHYDRATE	CARBOHYDRATE (OF WHICH SUGARS)	PROTEIN	FIBRE
100	5g	0.7g	14g	9g	2g	4g

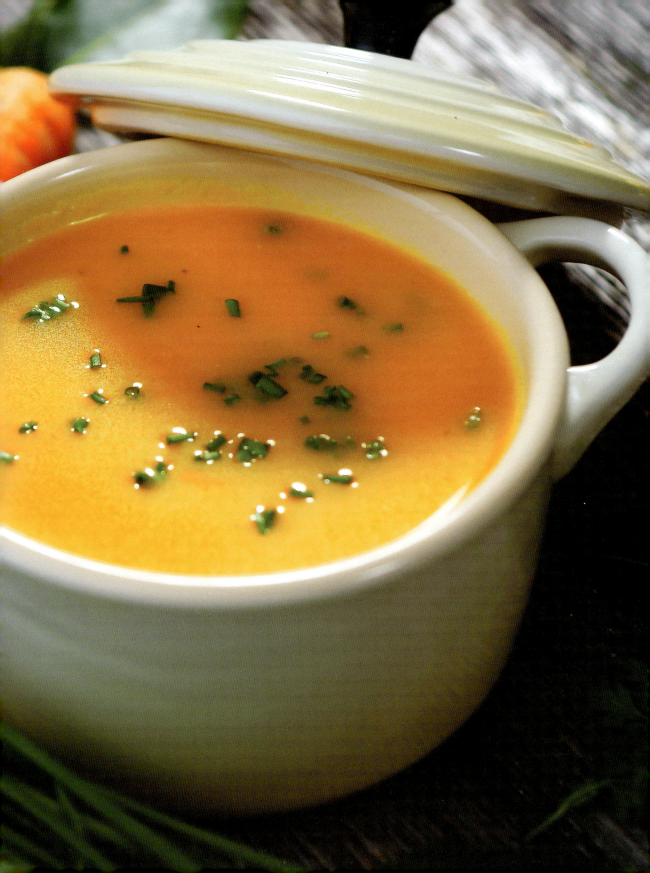

Carrot and coriander soup

Serves: 4–5 (makes 1.6l) **Prep time:** 10 mins **Cooking time:** 30 mins

Ingredients

- 4 tsp. olive oil or rapeseed oil
- 2 onions, chopped
- 2 cloves garlic, crushed
- 1 tsp. ground coriander
- 1 potato, peeled and cubed
- 6 carrots, peeled and chopped
- Freshly ground black pepper
- 1800ml/7½ cups vegetable stock
- 2 tsp. chopped coriander
- 2 tsp. honey
- Pepper to season

Method

1. Heat the oil in a large pot on a medium heat, add the onion and sauté until soft.

2. Add the garlic, coriander, potatoes and carrots and toss until well coated. Season with freshly ground black pepper.

3. Pour in the stock and bring to the boil. Lower the heat and simmer for 20 minutes until the vegetables are tender.

4. Blend with a hand blender.

5. Add the coriander and honey and serve hot.

NUTRITION INFORMATION
Amount per serving

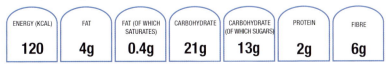

ENERGY (KCAL)	FAT	FAT (OF WHICH SATURATES)	CARBOHYDRATE	CARBOHYDRATE (OF WHICH SUGARS)	PROTEIN	FIBRE
120	4g	0.4g	21g	13g	2g	6g

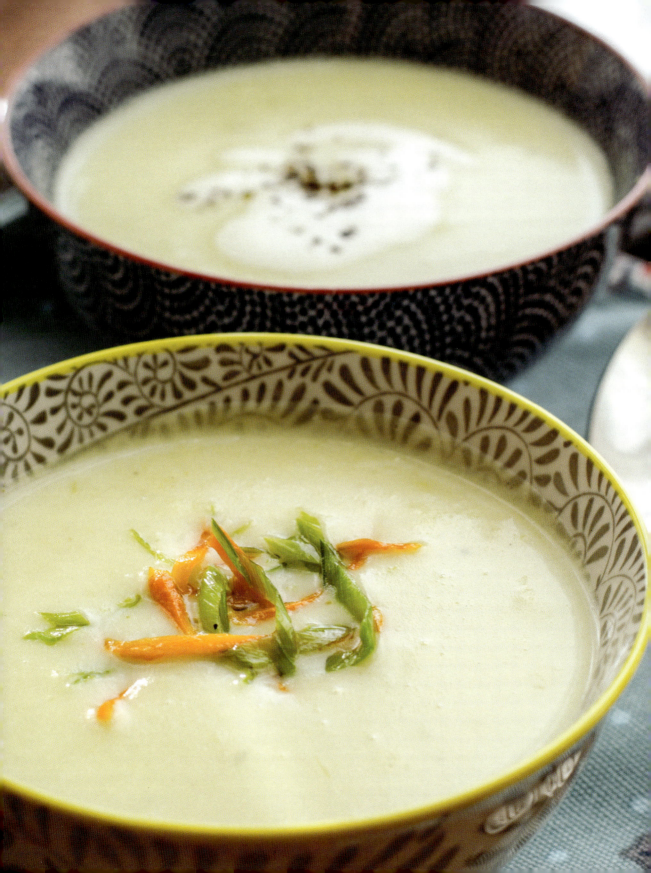

Chicken and vegetable soup

🍽 **Serves:** 7 (makes 2.5l) ⏱ **Prep time:** 10 mins ♨ **Cooking time:** <1 hour

Ingredients

- 1000ml/4¼ cups water
- 4 chicken breasts
- 1 tbsp. olive oil
- 1 large onion, peeled and chopped
- 1 small leek, peeled and chopped
- 2 celery stalks, chopped
- 2 small potatoes, peeled and chopped
- 4 medium carrots, peeled and chopped
- 1 bay leaf
- 200ml/1 cup of milk
- 1 tbsp. chopped fresh parsley
- 1 tbsp. chopped chives
- Freshly ground black pepper

Method

1. Poach the chicken in the water for 20 minutes. Remove chicken and shred with 2 forks. Keep the water to use as stock.

2. Heat the oil in a large saucepan over a medium heat and gently fry the onion, celery and leek for about 10 minutes.

3. Add in the carrot and potato, cook for 5 minutes.

4. Add the reserved water from cooking the chicken and bring the mixture to the boil, stirring as you do so. Add the bay leaf and then reduce the heat until the mixture is simmering. Simmer for approximately 30 minutes, until the vegetables are tender.

5. Remove the bay leaf, then, using a stick blender, blend the vegetables.

6. Add the milk and cooked chicken and cook until heated through. Season with freshly ground black pepper and stir in the parsley and chives and serve.

NUTRITION INFORMATION
Amount per serving

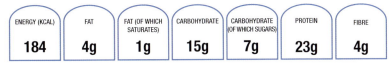

ENERGY (KCAL)	FAT	FAT (OF WHICH SATURATES)	CARBOHYDRATE	CARBOHYDRATE (OF WHICH SUGARS)	PROTEIN	FIBRE
184	4g	1g	15g	7g	23g	4g

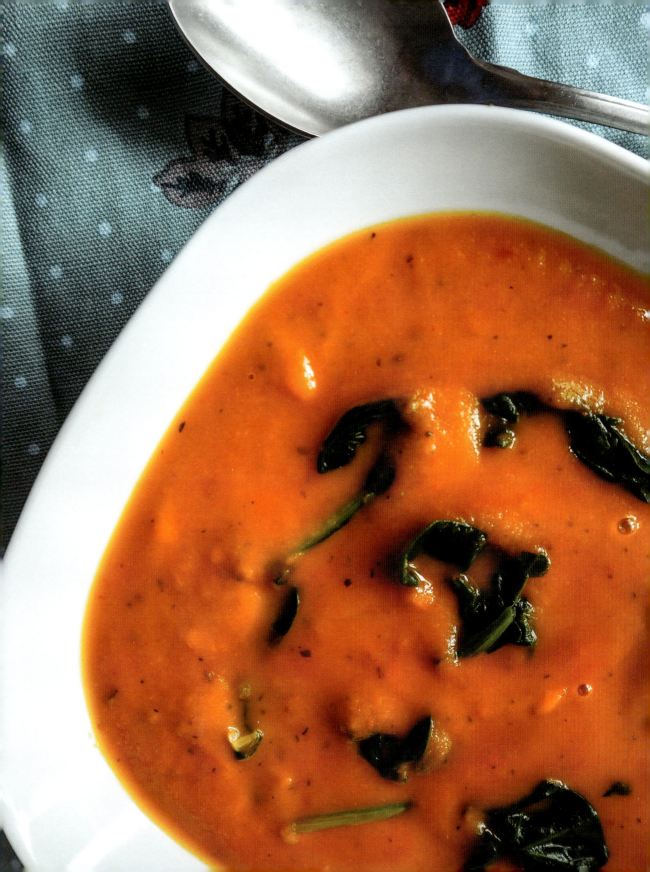

Lentil and spinach soup

🍽 **Serves:** 4–5 (makes 1.6l) ⏱ **Prep time:** 15 mins 🍲 **Cooking time:** 45 mins

Ingredients

- 2 tsp. olive oil
- 1 medium onion, finely chopped
- 2 garlic cloves, finely chopped
- 2 small sticks of celery, finely chopped
- 2 large carrots, finely chopped
- ½ tsp. chilli powder
- 1 tsp. smoked paprika
- 1 tsp. cumin seeds
- 200g/1 cup red lentils, washed
- 1700ml/7 cups vegetable stock
- 50g/¼ cup spinach, stalks removed and roughly chopped
- 100g/½ cup cherry tomatoes, halved

Method

1. Heat the oil in a large saucepan over a medium heat. Add the onion, garlic, celery and carrots and cook for 4–5 minutes or until starting to soften.

2. Add the chilli powder, paprika and cumin seeds and cook for 1 minute, stirring occasionally.

3. Add the red lentils and stock, bring to the boil, then cook for 10 minutes. Cover and reduce the heat to low, then simmer gently for 20–25 minutes, or until the vegetables and lentils are cooked.

4. Add the spinach and tomatoes and cook for 5 minutes more or until the spinach has wilted. Blend and serve.

NUTRITION INFORMATION
Amount per serving

ENERGY (KCAL)	FAT	FAT (OF WHICH SATURATES)	CARBOHYDRATE	CARBOHYDRATE (OF WHICH SUGARS)	PROTEIN	FIBRE
170	2g	0.3g	29g	6g	11g	5g

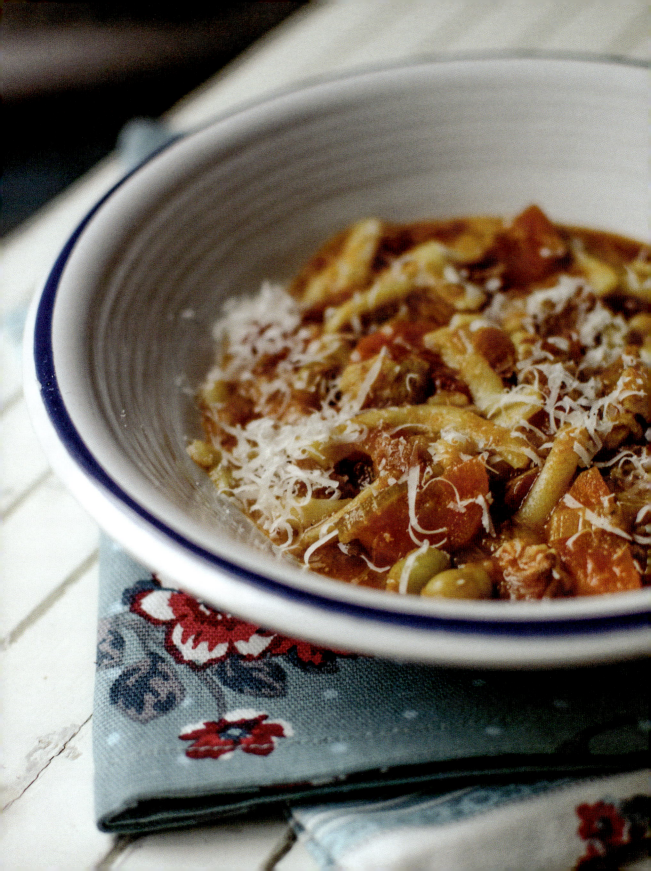

Minestrone

🍽 **Serves:** 7 (make 2.5l) ⏱ **Prep time:** 15 mins 🍲 **Cooking time:** 40 mins

Ingredients

- 1 tbsp. olive oil
- 1 large red onion, peeled and chopped
- 4 cloves garlic, chopped
- 2 carrots, chopped
- 2 small sticks of celery, chopped
- 2 x 400g/14oz tins of tomatoes
- 1000ml/4¼ cups vegetable stock
- 100g/1 cup wholewheat pasta, any shape
- 1 tin butter beans, drained
- Freshly ground black pepper
- 2 tsp. honey
- 2 handfuls of frozen peas
- 20g/1 cup fresh basil

Method

1. Heat the oil in a large pot and sauté the onion, garlic, carrots, and celery for 5 minutes.

2. Add the tomatoes to the pot and bring to the boil for 5 minutes.

3. Add in the stock, beans and pepper. Turn down the heat and simmer for 30 minutes.

4. Add the pasta and cook for 10–12 minutes until it is cooked through.

5. Add the honey and peas and cook for a further 2 minutes.

6. Add the basil and serve.

NUTRITION INFORMATION
Amount per serving

ENERGY (KCAL)	FAT	FAT (OF WHICH SATURATES)	CARBOHYDRATE	CARBOHYDRATE (OF WHICH SUGARS)	PROTEIN	FIBRE
148	3g	0.4g	25g	11g	6g	6g

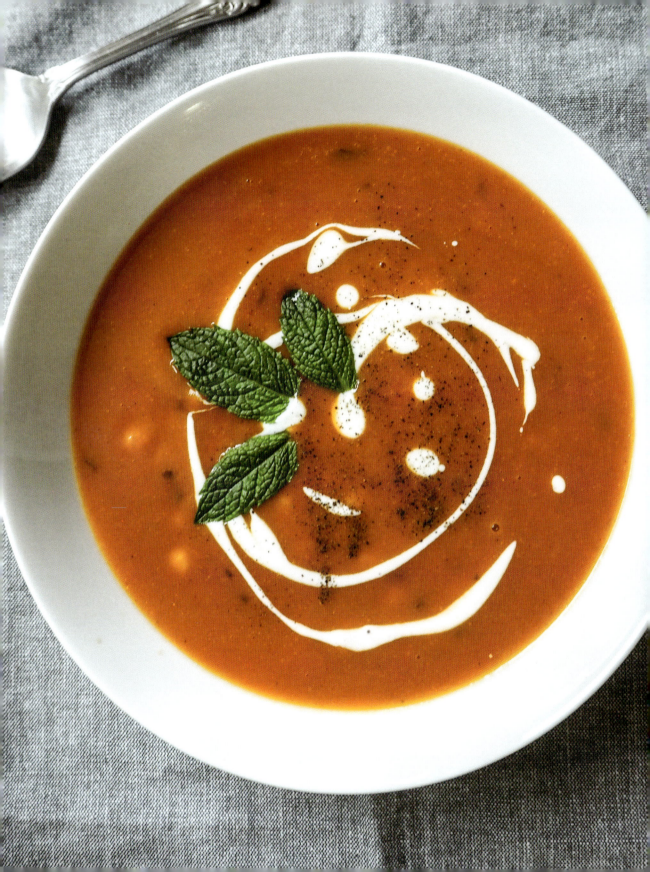

Moroccan roasted vegetable and chickpea soup

🍽 **Serves:** 7 (make 2.4l) ⏱ **Prep time:** 15 mins 🍲 **Cooking time:** 45 mins

Ingredients

- 1 large red onion, cut into wedges
- 3 carrots, peeled and cut into cubes
- 2 parsnips, peeled and cut into cubes
- ½ butternut squash, peeled and cut into cubes
- 1 small potato, peeled and cut into cubes
- 2 garlic cloves, crushed
- 1½ tbsp. olive oil
- 2 tsp. cumin
- 1 tsp. coriander
- ½ tsp. cinnamon
- ½ tsp. turmeric
- 1 tin chickpeas, drained
- 1300ml/5½ cups vegetable stock
- To serve: 1 tsp. low-fat Greek yogurt and fresh mint
- Freshly ground black pepper

Method

1. Preheat the oven to 200°C/400°F (fan 180°C/350°F) or gas mark 6. Lay the vegetables out in a roasting tin, coat with the spices and oil and mix well.

2. Roast for 30–35 minutes, mixing half way through to ensure even cooking.

3. Transfer the roasted vegetables to a large saucepan, add the chickpeas, pour over the hot stock and simmer for 5 minutes.

4. Blend the soup until smooth, then serve with yogurt, fresh mint and black pepper.

NUTRITION INFORMATION
Amount per serving

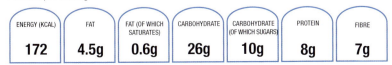

ENERGY (KCAL)	FAT	FAT (OF WHICH SATURATES)	CARBOHYDRATE	CARBOHYDRATE (OF WHICH SUGARS)	PROTEIN	FIBRE
172	4.5g	0.6g	26g	10g	8g	7g

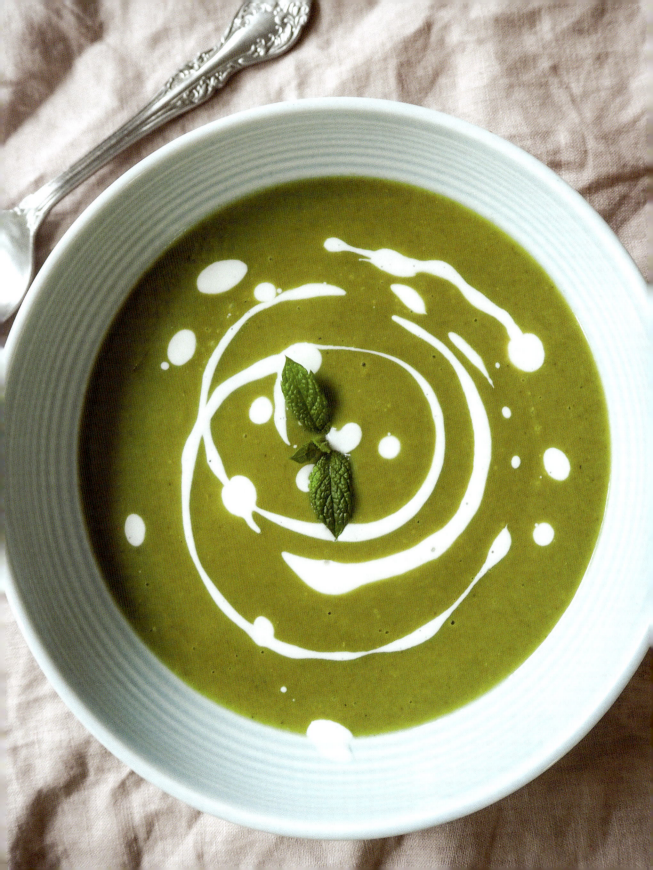

Pea and mint soup

🍽 **Serves:** 5–6 (makes 2l) ⏱ **Prep time:** 10 mins 🍲 **Cooking time:** 20 mins

Ingredients

- 1 bunch spring onions, trimmed and roughly chopped
- 1 medium potato, peeled and diced
- 1 garlic clove, peeled and crushed
- 850ml/3½ cups vegetable or chicken stock
- 900g/2lb frozen peas
- 3 tbsp. chopped fresh mint
- Large pinch caster sugar
- 1 tbsp. fresh lemon or lime juice
- 150ml/¾ cup sour cream

Method

1. Put the spring onions into a large pan with the potato, garlic and stock. Bring to the boil, turn down the heat and simmer for 15 minutes or until the potato is very soft.

2. Add the peas to the pot and simmer for another 5 minutes.

3. Stir in the mint, sugar and lemon or lime juice. Allow to cool before blending until smooth. Stir in half of the sour cream and season to taste.

4. The soup can be served cold or hot. If reheating, avoid boiling the soup after the sour cream has been added.

5. Serve the soup garnished with a drizzle of sour cream.

NUTRITION INFORMATION
Amount per serving

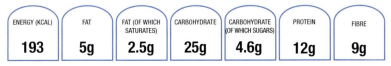

ENERGY (KCAL)	FAT	FAT (OF WHICH SATURATES)	CARBOHYDRATE	CARBOHYDRATE (OF WHICH SUGARS)	PROTEIN	FIBRE
193	5g	2.5g	25g	4.6g	12g	9g

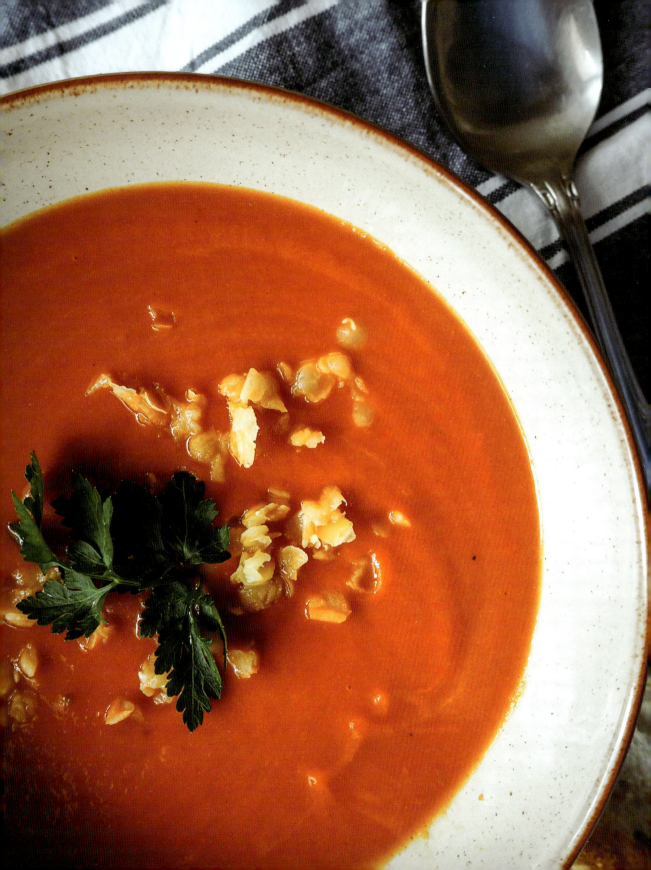

Red lentil and tomato soup

🍽 **Serves:** 6 (makes 2l) ⏱ **Prep time:** 5 mins 🍲 **Cooking time:** 30 mins

Ingredients

- 1½ tbsp. olive oil
- 2 medium onions, chopped
- 3–4 cloves of garlic, chopped
- 180g/¾ cup red lentils, rinsed under cold running water
- 1 x 400g/14oz tin chopped tomatoes
- 1800ml/7½ cups vegetable stock
- Pinch of nutmeg
- 2 tsp. honey
- Black pepper to season

Method

1. Fry the chopped onion and crushed garlic in the olive oil until the onion begins to soften, about 5 minutes.

2. Add the lentils and stir until the lentils have absorbed the oil.

3. Add the tin of tomatoes and heat the mixture through.

4. Add the stock and bring to the boil.

5. Simmer for 15–20 minutes until the lentils are breaking up. Blend and season with honey, nutmeg and pepper.

NUTRITION INFORMATION
Amount per serving

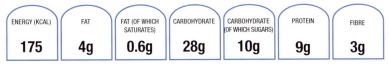

ENERGY (KCAL)	FAT	FAT (OF WHICH SATURATES)	CARBOHYDRATE	CARBOHYDRATE (OF WHICH SUGARS)	PROTEIN	FIBRE
175	4g	0.6g	28g	10g	9g	3g

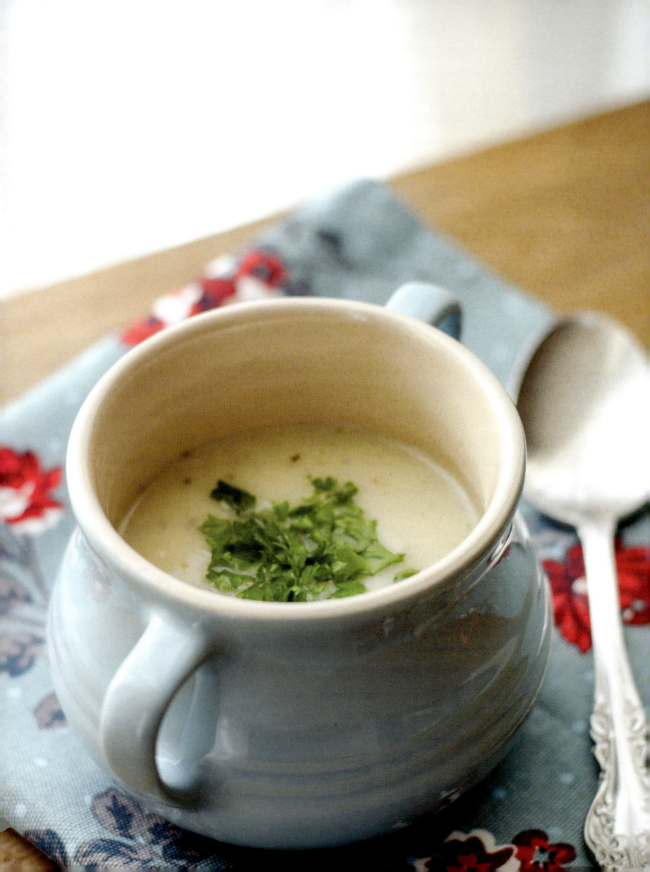

Roast chicken soup

Serves: 5–6 (makes 2l) **Prep time:** 15 mins **Cooking time:** 35 mins

Ingredients

- 1 tbsp. olive oil
- 2 medium onions, chopped
- 3 medium carrots, chopped
- 1 garlic clove, crushed
- 1 tsp. thyme leaves
- 1.4l/6 cups chicken stock
- 300g/11oz leftover roast chicken, shredded and skin removed
- 200g/1$^1/_3$ cups frozen peas
- Freshly ground black pepper
- 3 tbsp. Greek yogurt
- Squeeze lemon juice

Method

1. Heat oil in a large heavy-based pan. Add the onions, carrots, garlic and thyme. Cover and cook gently for 15 minutes.

2. Stir in the stock, bring to a boil, cover, then simmer for 10 minutes.

3. Add the chicken. Remove half the mixture, then puree with a stick blender.

4. Tip back into the pan with the rest of the soup, peas and seasoning, then simmer for 5 minutes until heated through.

5. Mix the yogurt and lemon juice, swirl into the soup in bowls, then serve.

NUTRITION INFORMATION
Amount per serving

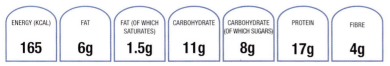

ENERGY (KCAL)	FAT	FAT (OF WHICH SATURATES)	CARBOHYDRATE	CARBOHYDRATE (OF WHICH SUGARS)	PROTEIN	FIBRE
165	6g	1.5g	11g	8g	17g	4g

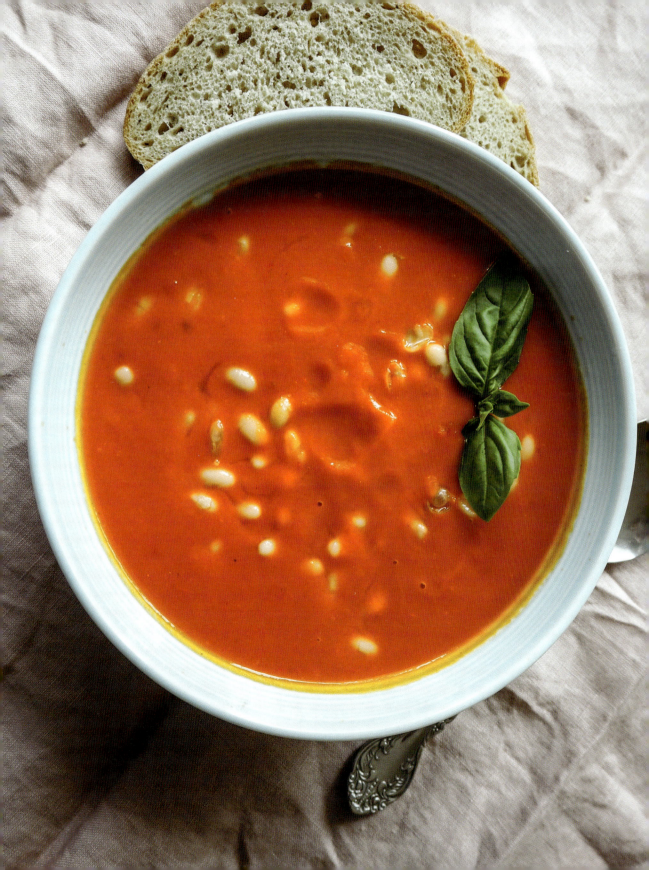

Tomato and cannellini bean soup

🍽 **Serves:** 5 (1.6l) ⏱ **Prep time:** 5 mins 🍲 **Cooking time:** 5 mins

Ingredients

- 2 tsp. olive oil
- 1 onion, finely chopped
- 600g/3 cups fresh whole tomatoes, quartered
- ½ red chilli, finely chopped
- 1 x 400g/14oz tin chopped tomatoes
- 500ml/2 cups vegetable stock
- Handful basil leaves
- 400g/14oz tin cannellini beans, drained and rinsed

Method

1. Heat the olive oil in a large pan over a medium heat. Add the onion and cook for about 5 minutes, until softened.

2. Stir in the fresh tomatoes and chilli. Cover and cook for 10 minutes, stirring occasionally.

3. Add the tinned tomatoes and stock to the pan and stir well. Bring to the boil, then cover and simmer for 20 minutes, stirring occasionally.

4. Add the beans and heat through.

5. Take the pan off the heat and stir in the basil. Puree the soup with a hand blender until smooth.

NUTRITION INFORMATION
Amount per serving

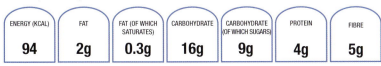

ENERGY (KCAL)	FAT	FAT (OF WHICH SATURATES)	CARBOHYDRATE	CARBOHYDRATE (OF WHICH SUGARS)	PROTEIN	FIBRE
94	2g	0.3g	16g	9g	4g	5g

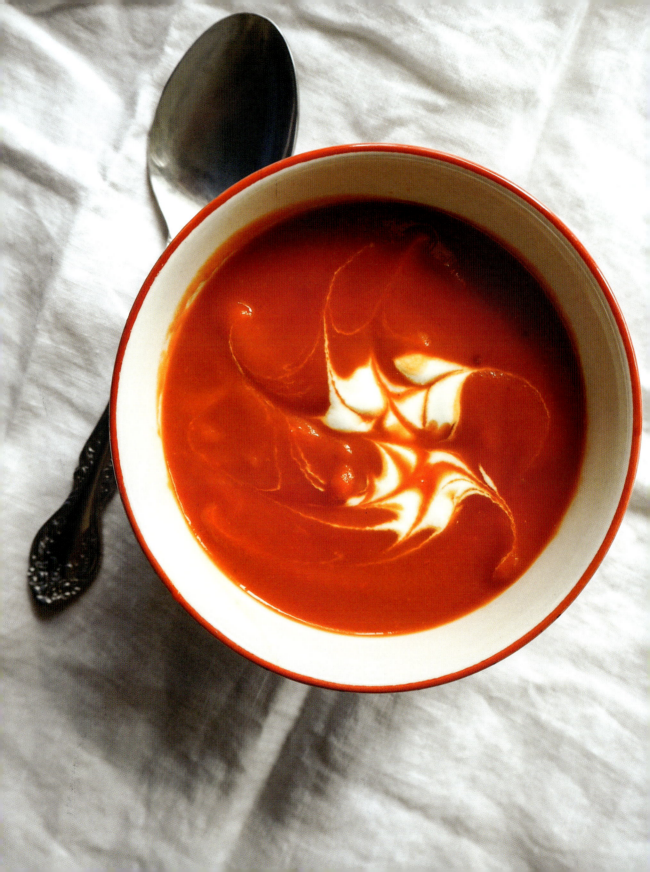

Tomato and roasted red pepper soup

🍽 **Serves:** 4 (makes 1.6l) ⏱ **Prep time:** 5 mins 🍲 **Cooking time:** 40 mins

Ingredients

- 2 red peppers
- 1 onion, peeled and chopped
- 1 tbsp. olive oil
- 2 garlic cloves, peeled and finely chopped
- 1 tsp. tomato puree
- Pinch ground cinnamon
- 750ml/3¼ cups vegetable or chicken stock
- 1 x 400g/14oz tin of chopped tomatoes
- Sprig of thyme
- Freshly ground black pepper
- Pinch of sugar
- 1 tsp. lime juice
- Half-fat/reduced-fat crème fraiche to serve

Method

1. Grill the red peppers under the grill until charred. Transfer to a bowl, cover with cling film and leave to cool. Deseed, remove the skins and roughly chop.

2. Sauté the onion in olive oil for about 5 minutes, until translucent. Add the garlic, cinnamon and tomato puree and cook for 2 minutes.

3. Then add the stock, tomatoes, thyme and some black pepper.

4. Bring to the boil, reduce the heat and simmer for 20 minutes.

5. Stir in the roasted peppers and sugar and remove from the heat. Puree the soup in a blender.

6. Gently reheat once pureed, add the lime juice and season to taste. Serve with a dollop of crème fraiche if desired.

NUTRITION INFORMATION
Amount per serving

ENERGY (KCAL)	FAT	FAT (OF WHICH SATURATES)	CARBOHYDRATE	CARBOHYDRATE (OF WHICH SUGARS)	PROTEIN	FIBRE
105	6g	2g	12g	10g	2g	3g

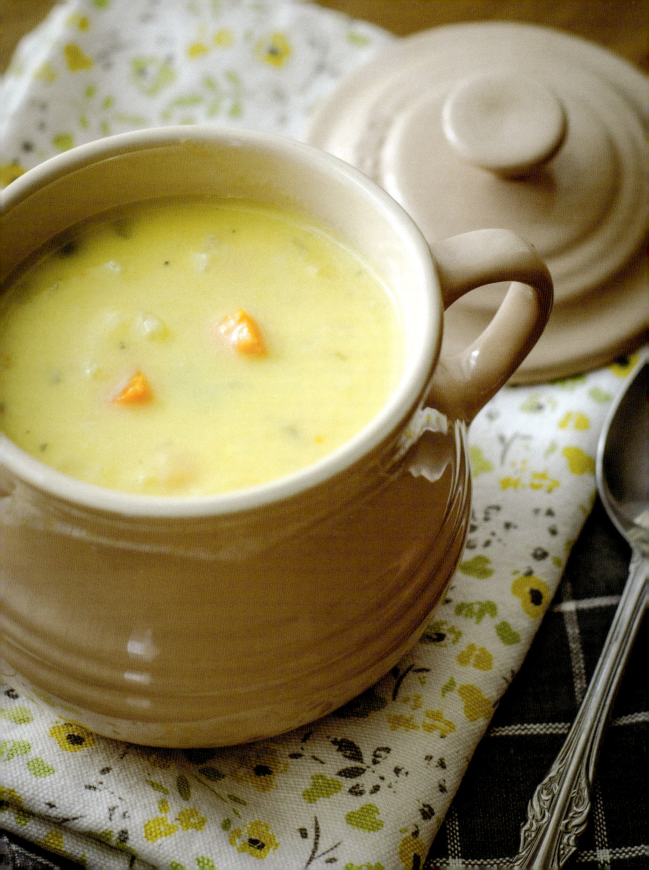

Vegetable soup

🍽 **Serves:** 7 (makes 2.4l) ⏱ **Prep time:** 10 mins 🍲 **Cooking time:** 30 mins

Ingredients

- 1 tbsp. olive oil
- 1 large onion, peeled and chopped
- 1 leek, chopped
- 2 carrots, peeled and chopped
- 3 sticks celery, chopped
- ½ turnip or ¼ celeriac, peeled and chopped
- 1 potato, peeled and cut in cubes
- Fresh thyme
- 1.4l/6 cups stock
- Low-fat milk to finish
- Fresh parsley, finely chopped
- Freshly ground black pepper to season

Method

1. Heat the oil and sauté the onion and leek for 5 minutes in a covered pan.

2. Add in the remaining vegetables and thyme and cook for 10 minutes.

3. Add the stock and simmer for 20–30 minutes until the vegetables are soft. Blend soup with a splash of milk.

4. Check the seasoning and finish with finely chopped parsley.

NUTRITION INFORMATION
Amount per serving

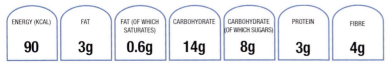

ENERGY (KCAL)	FAT	FAT (OF WHICH SATURATES)	CARBOHYDRATE	CARBOHYDRATE (OF WHICH SUGARS)	PROTEIN	FIBRE
90	3g	0.6g	14g	8g	3g	4g

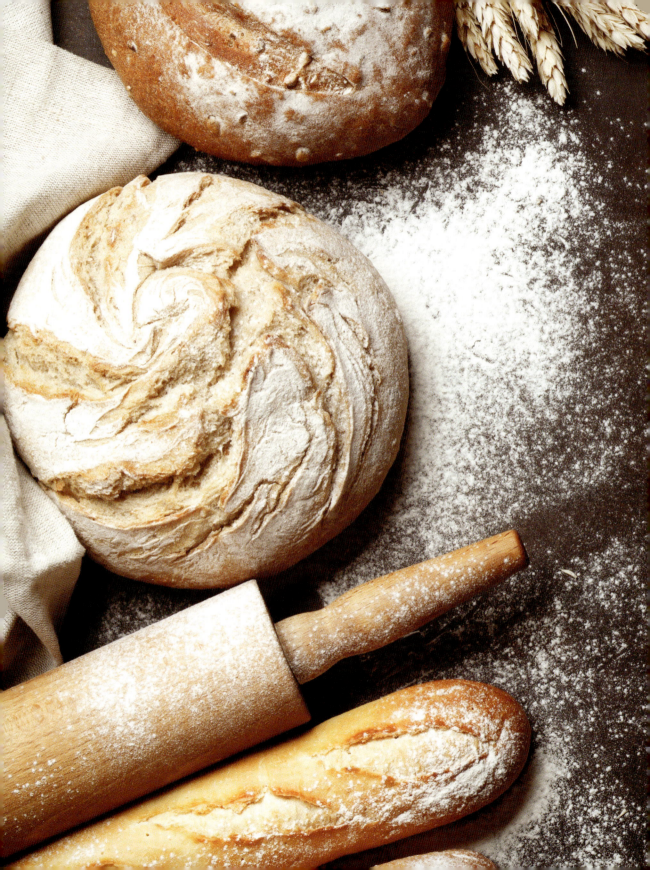

Bread

——

Oat bread

Soda bread

Brown bread with seeds

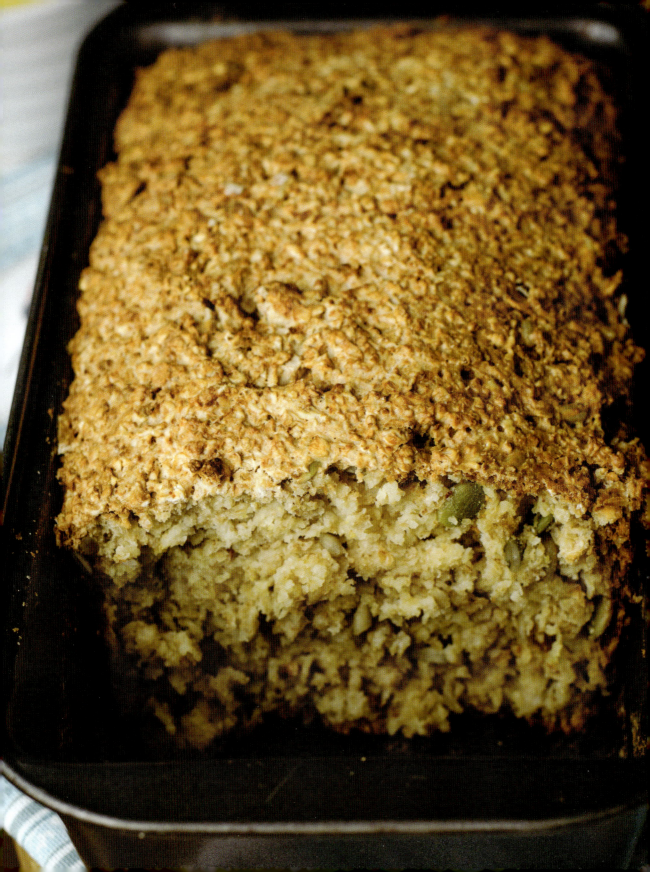

Oat bread

🍽 **Serves:** Makes 1 loaf ⏱ **Prep time:** 10 mins 🍲 **Cooking time:** 1 hour

Ingredients

- 500g/2 cups low-fat natural yogurt
- 3–4 tbsp. milk
- 1 egg
- 2 tsp. bicarbonate of soda
- 500g/5 cups porridge oats
- ½ tsp. salt

Method

1. Preheat the oven to 180°C/350°F (fan 160°C/320°F) or gas mark 4. Line a standard loaf tin (2lb) using parchment paper.

2. In a mixing bowl combine the yogurt, milk, egg and bicarbonate of soda.

3. Stir in the oats and salt. Ensure all ingredients are well blended into a doughy texture and then transfer the mixture to the loaf tin.

4. Cut a line down the centre of your loaf and place in the oven and cook for 45–55 minutes (shorter time for fan-assisted ovens).

5. Remove the loaf from the tin. Return to the oven upside down and allow to cook for 5 minutes more to make loaf crispy.

6. Insert a skewer to ensure that the inside of the loaf is cooked before removing from the oven.

7. Leave to cool on a wire tray.

NUTRITION INFORMATION
Amount per serving

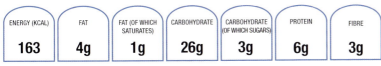

ENERGY (KCAL)	FAT	FAT (OF WHICH SATURATES)	CARBOHYDRATE	CARBOHYDRATE (OF WHICH SUGARS)	PROTEIN	FIBRE
163	4g	1g	26g	3g	6g	3g

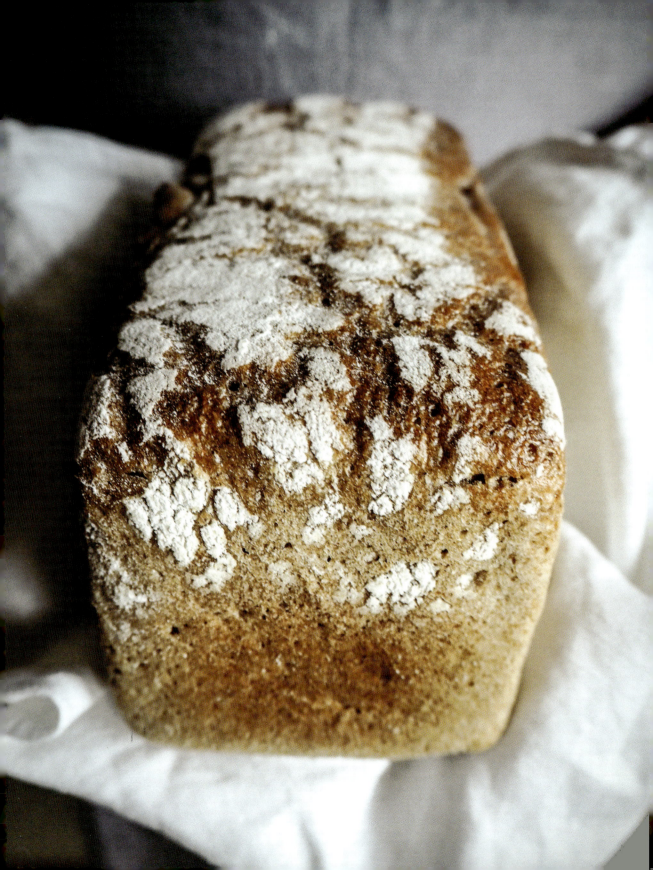

Soda bread

Serves: Makes 1 loaf **Prep time:** 10 mins **Cooking time:** 1 hour

Ingredients

- 300ml/1¼ cups semi-skimmed milk
- 1 tbsp. lemon juice
- 225g/1¾ cups plain flour
- ½ tsp. salt
- 1 tsp. bicarbonate of soda
- 225g/1¾ cups wholemeal flour
- 1 tsp. sugar

Method

1. Mix the milk and lemon juice and leave to stand for 5 minutes to sour the milk.

2. Preheat the oven to 200°C/400°F (fan 180°C/350°F) or gas mark 6.

3. In a large bowl, sift the white flour, salt and bicarbonate of soda, then add the wholemeal flour and sugar and mix. Then add the soured milk, a little at a time, mixing continuously to make a firm dough.

4. Turn the dough into a greased 2lb loaf tin.

5. Place in the oven and bake for 15 minutes, then reduce the temperature to 180°C/350°F (fan 160°C/320°F) or gas mark 4 and cook for a further 45 minutes.

NUTRITION INFORMATION
Amount per serving

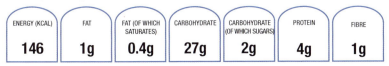

ENERGY (KCAL)	FAT	FAT (OF WHICH SATURATES)	CARBOHYDRATE	CARBOHYDRATE (OF WHICH SUGARS)	PROTEIN	FIBRE
146	1g	0.4g	27g	2g	4g	1g

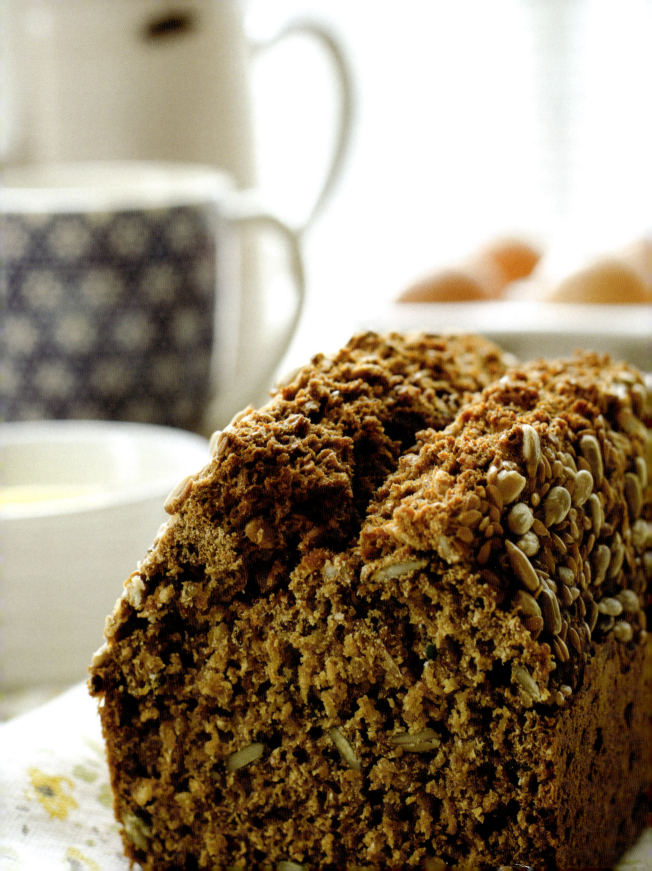

Brown bread with seeds

🍽 **Serves:** Makes 1 loaf ⏱ **Prep time:** 10 mins 🍲 **Cooking time:** 45 mins

Ingredients

- 400g/3^1/$_3$ cups brown flour
- 100g/¾ cup white flour
- 25g/½ cup bran
- 50g/^{1}/$_3$ cup mixed seeds
- 1 level tsp. bread soda
- 1 egg
- 1 tbsp. olive oil or rapeseed oil
- 1 tsp. treacle
- 425ml/1¾ cups buttermilk

Method

1. Place the dry ingredients in a bowl.

2. Mix the oil, egg, treacle and buttermilk together.

3. Add the wet ingredients to the dry and mix well.

4. Place in a greased loaf tin.

5. Bake at 200°C/400°F (fan 180°C/350°F) or gas mark 6 for 45 minutes.

NUTRITION INFORMATION
Amount per serving

ENERGY (KCAL)	FAT	FAT (OF WHICH SATURATES)	CARBOHYDRATE	CARBOHYDRATE (OF WHICH SUGARS)	PROTEIN	FIBRE
165	3g	0.6g	27g	2g	7g	3g

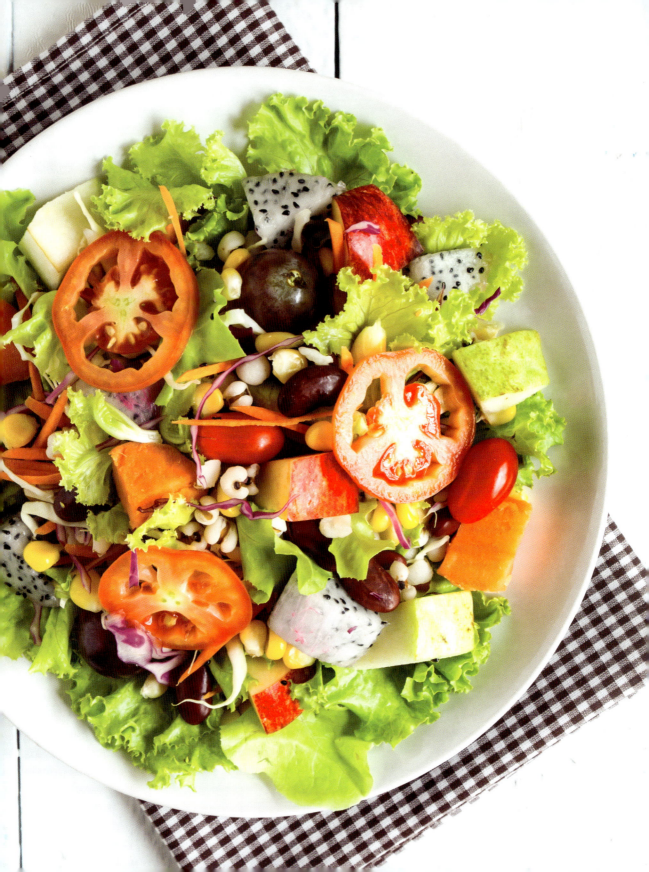

Salads

Crunchy tossed salad

Chickpea and mango salad

Salmon and pasta salad

Italian salad

Quinoa with roasted vegetables and feta

Three-grain salad

Quick salad with berries

Warm chicken salad with French dressing

Warm shredded chicken and chilli salad

Rainbow salad

Pink tabbouleh salad

Roast squash, bean and kale salad

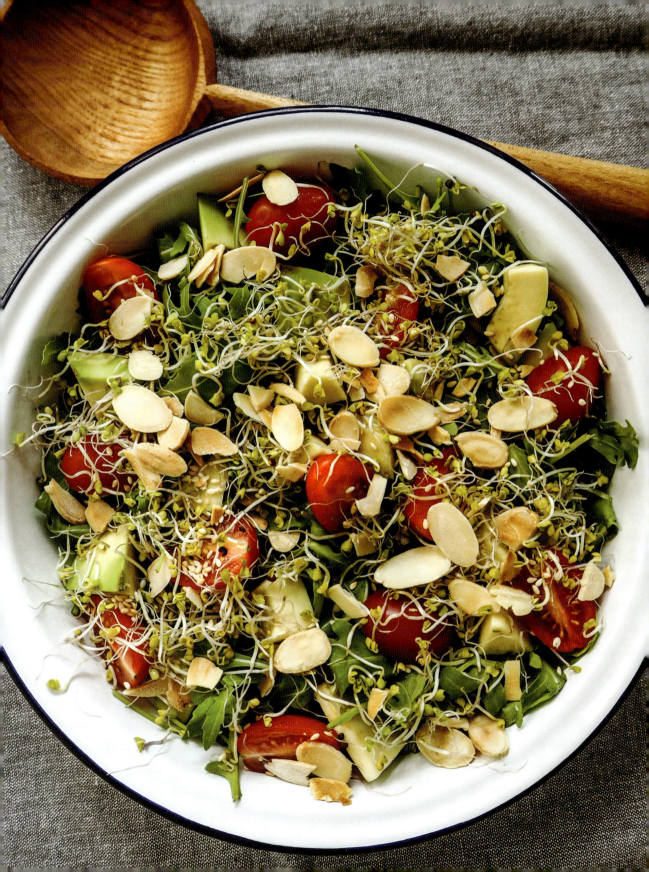

Crunchy tossed salad

🍽 **Serves:** 2 ⏱ **Prep time:** 10 mins

Ingredients

- 100g/3½oz fresh rocket
- 6–8 cherry tomatoes, halved
- 1 ripe avocado
- 80g/½ cup bean sprouts
- 50g/½ cup toasted almond flakes
- 1 heaped tbsp. toasted sesame seeds

For the dressing:
- 1 clove garlic
- Juice ½ lemon
- A drizzle of olive oil

Method

1. Put the rocket and tomatoes in a bowl.

2. Cut the avocado in half, remove the stone and score through the flesh in each half, up and down and then across, making sure not to cut through the skin. Scrape the pieces into the bowl.

3. Add the sprouts, flaked almonds and sesame seeds.

4. Finely chop the garlic, then mix all the dressing ingredients in a mug and pour over the salad.

5. Mix well and enjoy.

NUTRITION INFORMATION
Amount per serving

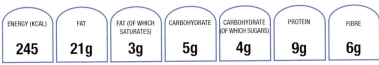

ENERGY (KCAL)	FAT	FAT (OF WHICH SATURATES)	CARBOHYDRATE	CARBOHYDRATE (OF WHICH SUGARS)	PROTEIN	FIBRE
245	21g	3g	5g	4g	9g	6g

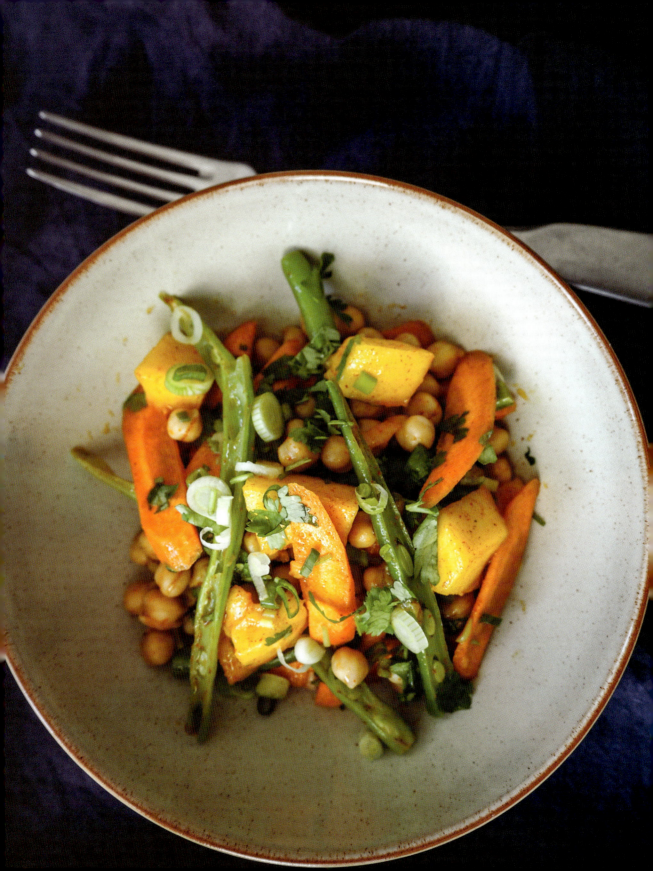

Chickpea and mango salad

🍽 **Serves:** 2 ⏱ **Prep time:** 10 mins

Ingredients

For the dressing:
- 3 scallions, trimmed
- ½ mango, peeled and chopped
- ½ tsp. paprika
- 3 tbsp. olive oil
- Juice of 1 lime

For the salad:
- 400g/14oz tin chickpeas, drained
- 2 carrots, peeled and finely sliced
- Handful green beans, sliced crossways
- 2 tbsp. finely chopped fresh coriander

Serve on a bed of mixed lettuce leaves (150g/3½oz).

Method

1. Place all of the ingredients for the dressing in a food processor and process until combined.

2. Place the chickpeas in a large serving bowl, tip in the mango dressing and stir to combine. Add the carrots and green beans and toss well. Sprinkle over the coriander to serve.

NUTRITION INFORMATION
Amount per serving

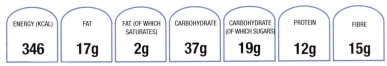

ENERGY (KCAL)	FAT	FAT (OF WHICH SATURATES)	CARBOHYDRATE	CARBOHYDRATE (OF WHICH SUGARS)	PROTEIN	FIBRE
346	17g	2g	37g	19g	12g	15g

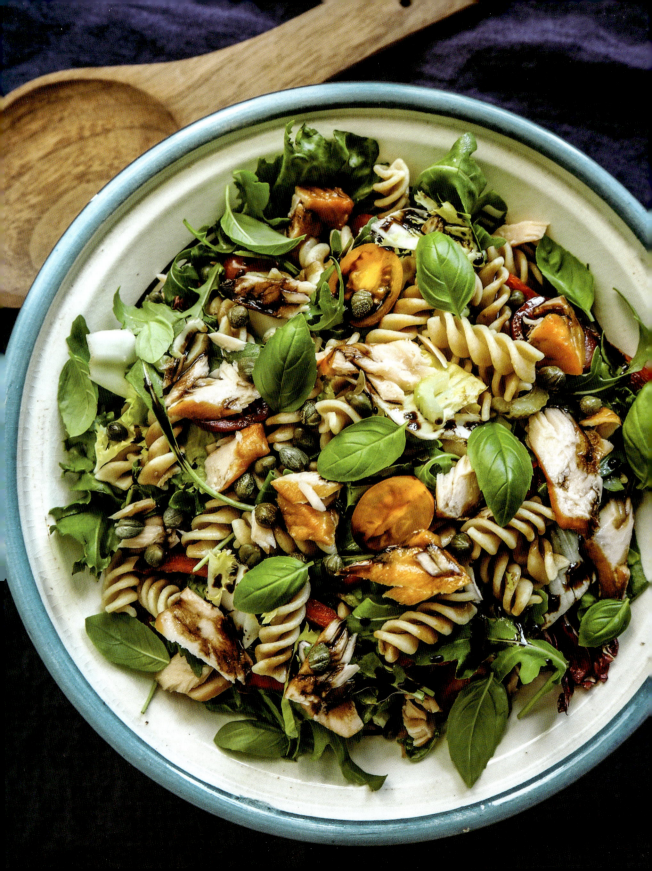

Salmon and pasta salad

🍽 **Serves:** 4 ⏱ **Prep time:** 20 mins 🍲 **Cooking time:** 10 mins

Ingredients

- 160g/1½ cups (raw) wholegrain pasta
- 225g/8oz tinned salmon, drained
- 1 tbsp. capers, drained
- 1 pepper, sliced
- 1 stick celery, sliced
- 250g/1¼ cups cherry tomatoes, halved
- 100g/3½oz rocket leaves
- 100g/3½oz mixed lettuce
- Handful of basil leaves
- 3 tbsp. extra virgin olive oil
- 5 tbsp. balsamic vinegar

Method

1. Cook the pasta according to the instructions on the packet, drain and rinse with cold water.

2. Add the remaining prepared ingredients to the pasta.

3. Toss the salad and decorate with fresh basil leaves.

NUTRITION INFORMATION
Amount per serving

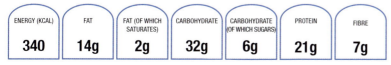

ENERGY (KCAL)	FAT	FAT (OF WHICH SATURATES)	CARBOHYDRATE	CARBOHYDRATE (OF WHICH SUGARS)	PROTEIN	FIBRE
340	14g	2g	32g	6g	21g	7g

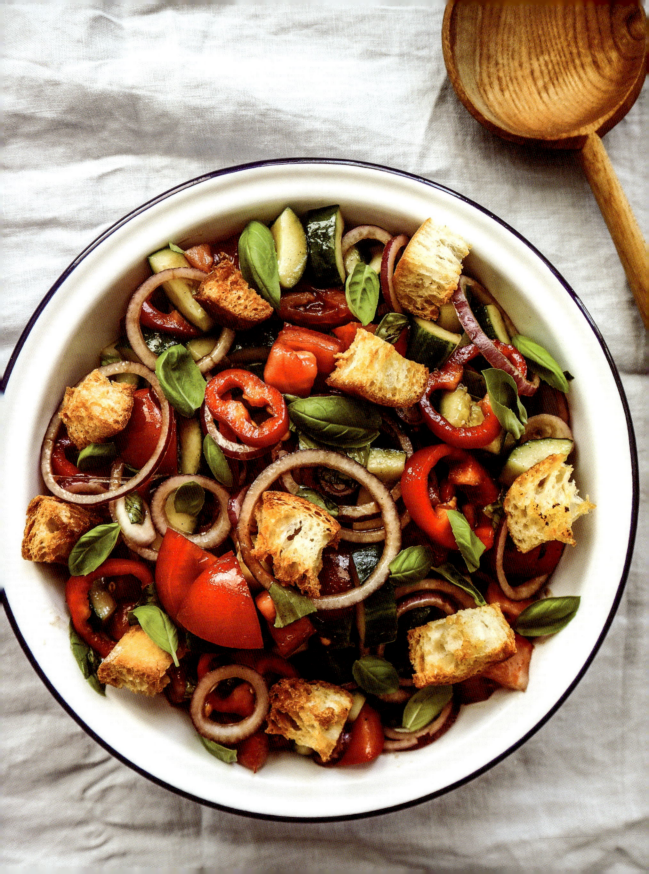

Italian salad

🍽 **Serves:** 4 ⏱ **Prep time:** 15 mins 🍲 **Cooking time:** 10 mins

Ingredients

- 4 ripe tomatoes, chopped
- Freshly ground black pepper
- 1 tbsp. capers, rinsed
- 1 sweet red pepper, sliced
- 1 cucumber, deseeded and chopped
- 1 red onion, finely sliced
- 2 garlic cloves, crushed
- 200g/7oz stale Italian bread, e.g. ciabatta
- 4 tbsp. olive oil
- 2 tbsp. balsamic vinegar
- 2 large handfuls of fresh basil

Method

1. Place the tomatoes in a bowl and season with freshly ground black pepper. Rinse the capers and add to the bowl, along with the pepper, cucumber, onion and garlic.

2. Tear or chop the stale ciabatta into cubes and spread them out on a lined baking tray. Spray with 1 kcal cooking spray and toast in a preheated oven at 200°C/400°F (fan 180°C/350°F) or gas mark 6 for a few minutes until brown.

3. Toss the mixture together with your hands, and then stir in the vinegar and olive oil. Taste and add a little more pepper, vinegar or oil, if needed.

4. Tear in the basil leaves, stir together and serve.

NUTRITION INFORMATION
Amount per serving

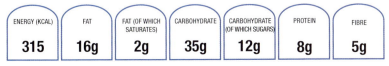

ENERGY (KCAL)	FAT	FAT (OF WHICH SATURATES)	CARBOHYDRATE	CARBOHYDRATE (OF WHICH SUGARS)	PROTEIN	FIBRE
315	16g	2g	35g	12g	8g	5g

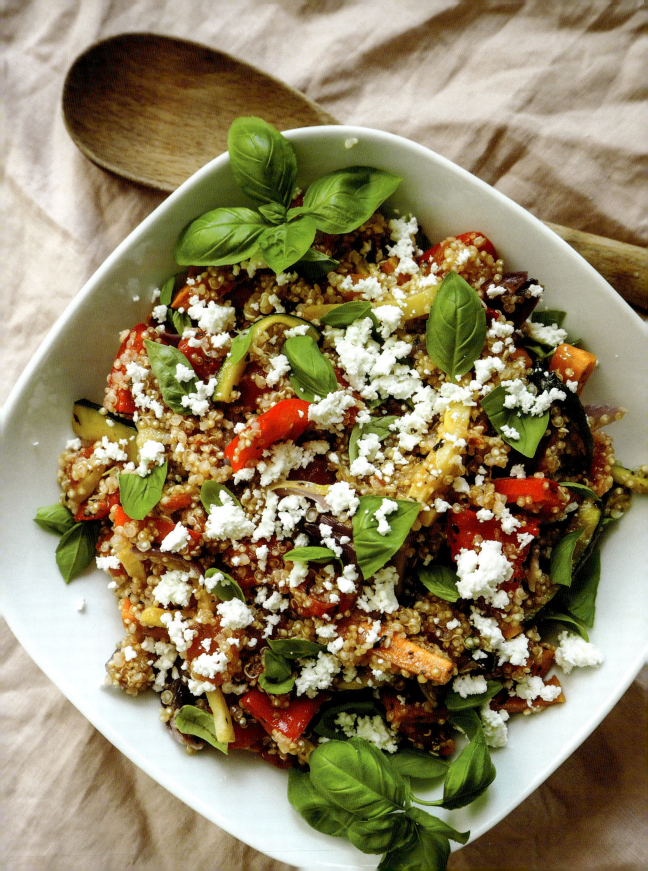

Quinoa with roasted vegetables and feta

🍽 **Serves:** 4–6 ⏱ **Prep time:** 20 mins 🍲 **Cooking time:** 25 mins

Ingredients

- 1 red onion, peeled and chopped into 1½cm/½in pieces
- 1 carrot, peeled and cut into 5cm/2in thin strips (julienne)
- 1 courgette, cut into 5cm/2in thin strips (julienne)
- 1 red pepper, chopped into 1½cm/½in pieces
- 2 cloves garlic, roughly chopped
- Pinch of dried oregano
- 2 tbsp. olive oil
- 1 x 400g/14oz tin chopped tomatoes
- 300g/1½cups quinoa (pre-cooked weight)
- 2 tbsp. fresh parsley, chopped
- 1 tbsp. fresh basil, chopped
- 200g/7oz feta cheese

Method

1. Preheat the oven to 220°C/425°F (fan 200°C/400°F) or gas mark 7.

2. Place the red onion, carrot, courgette and red pepper in an ovenproof dish. Add the garlic, a good pinch of dried oregano and olive oil. Toss well to coat all the vegetables.

3. Place on the top shelf of the preheated oven for 10 minutes. Remove from the oven and stir in the chopped tomatoes. Return to the oven for a further 15 minutes until the vegetables are soft.

4. Cook the quinoa as per packet instructions, strain and fluff it up with a fork. Place in a large bowl. Add the parsley and fresh basil. Mix well.

5. Stir in the roasted vegetables. Crumble the feta cheese on top and serve.

NUTRITION INFORMATION
Amount per serving

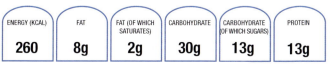

ENERGY (KCAL)	FAT	FAT (OF WHICH SATURATES)	CARBOHYDRATE	CARBOHYDRATE (OF WHICH SUGARS)	PROTEIN
260	8g	2g	30g	13g	13g

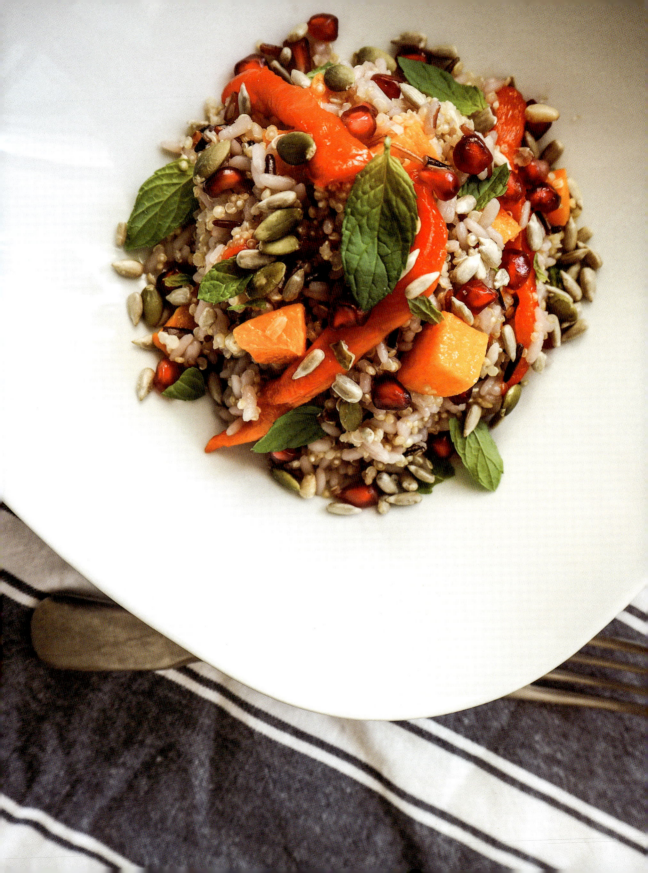

Three-grain salad

Serves: 6 Prep time: 10 mins Cooking time: 30 mins

Ingredients

- 1 butternut squash, peeled, deseeded, cubed
- 3 red peppers, chopped
- 1 tbsp. olive oil
- 100g/½ cup (pre-cooking weight) brown rice
- 100g/½ cup (pre-cooking weight) quinoa
- 100g/½ cup (pre-cooking weight) wild rice
- 1 pomegranate, seeds only
- 100g/⅔ cup seeds (pumpkin seeds and sunflower seeds)
- Handful of mint leaves
- 1 lemon, halved

Method

1. Heat the oven to 180°C/350°F (fan 160°C/320°F) or gas mark 4 and roast the squash and red peppers with 1 tbsp. of the oil for 30 minutes.

2. Cook the rice and quinoa in separate pots as per packet instructions.

3. Mix the rice, quinoa, red peppers and squash together and refrigerate immediately to cool.

4. When ready to serve, divide the salad between serving plates.

5. Toast the seeds in a dry pan for 3–4 minutes and sprinkle over the salad with the pomegranate seeds and the mint.

6. Squeeze over some lemon juice and serve.

NUTRITION INFORMATION
Amount per serving

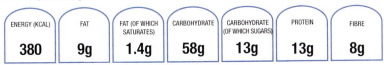

ENERGY (KCAL)	FAT	FAT (OF WHICH SATURATES)	CARBOHYDRATE	CARBOHYDRATE (OF WHICH SUGARS)	PROTEIN	FIBRE
380	9g	1.4g	58g	13g	13g	8g

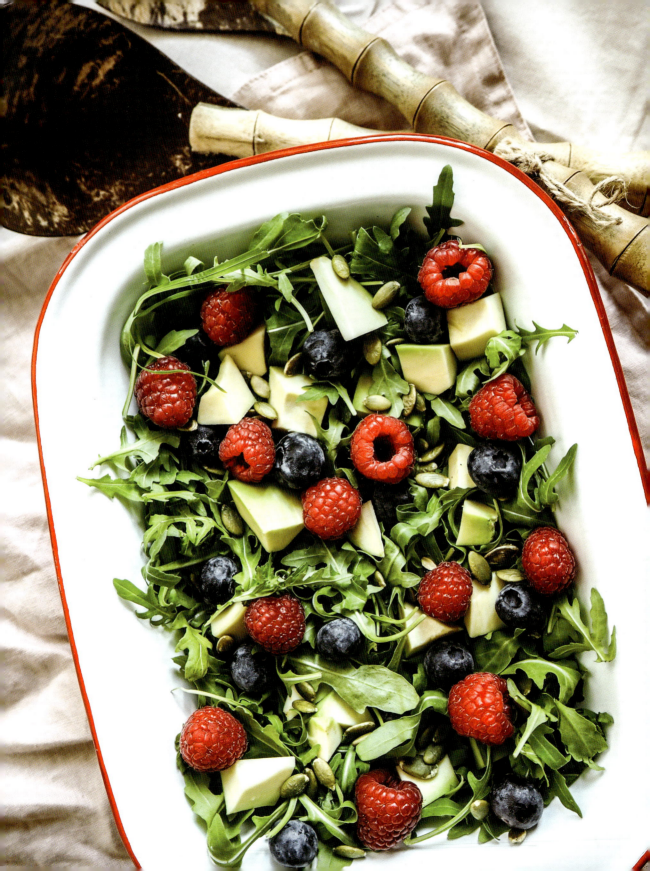

Quick salad with berries

🍽 **Serves:** 2 as a lunch/4 as a side ⏱ **Prep time:** 5 mins

Ingredients

- 80–100g/3–3½oz rocket or a similar green salad leaf, washed
- 1 ripe avocado
- Juice ½ lemon
- 2 tbsp. olive oil
- 2 tbsp. pumpkin seeds
- 125g/1 cup raspberries, washed
- 125g/1 cup blueberries, washed

Method

1. Place the rocket in a bowl.

2. Cut the avocado in half, then remove the stone and cut each half into small pieces, still in the skin, making sure not to cut through. Spoon out the flesh and add to the bowl of rocket.

3. Squeeze in the lemon juice, using your hand as a sieve to catch any pips, add olive oil and mix through.

4. Once the salad is dressed, add the seeds and top with the berries.

NUTRITION INFORMATION
Amount per serving

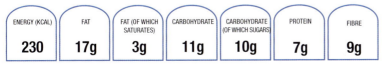

ENERGY (KCAL)	FAT	FAT (OF WHICH SATURATES)	CARBOHYDRATE	CARBOHYDRATE (OF WHICH SUGARS)	PROTEIN	FIBRE
230	17g	3g	11g	10g	7g	9g

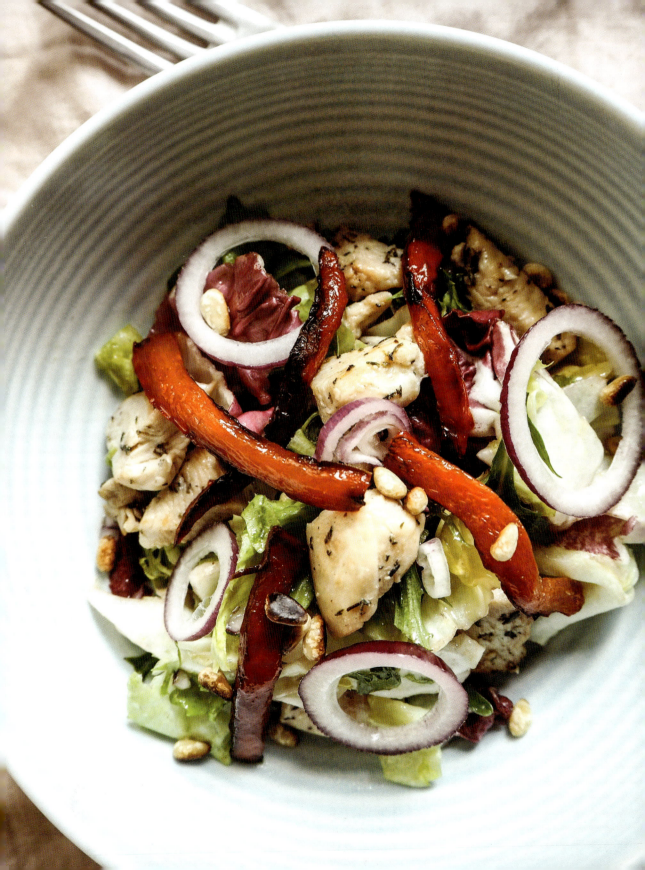

Warm chicken salad (with French dressing)

🍽 **Serves:** 2 ⏱ **Prep time:** 10 mins plus time for marinating

Ingredients

- 1 clove garlic, crushed
- ½ tsp. fresh thyme
- 1 red onion, finely sliced
- Salad leaves
- 2 tbsp. pine nuts, toasted
- 1 red pepper, roasted and skinned
- 2 cooked chicken fillets, chopped

French dressing (makes 8 servings)**:**
- 8 tbsp. oil (olive, sunflower or a mixture)
- 2 tbsp. white wine vinegar or lemon juice
- ½ tsp. honey/sugar
- 1 tsp. Dijon mustard
- Pepper

Method

1. Mix all of the dressing ingredients together and mix/shake well.

2. Mix the garlic and thyme with 2 tsp. of the French dressing. Add the chicken and allow to marinate (overnight if possible).

3. Mix the red onion with 1 tbsp. of French dressing. Leftover dressing can be stored in the fridge.

4. Dress the salad and add the red pepper, onion, pine nuts and cooked chicken.

NUTRITION INFORMATION
Amount per serving

ENERGY (KCAL)	FAT	FAT (OF WHICH SATURATES)	CARBOHYDRATE	CARBOHYDRATE (OF WHICH SUGARS)	PROTEIN	FIBRE
375.9	22.5g	3g	13.1g	10.6g	30.3g	3g

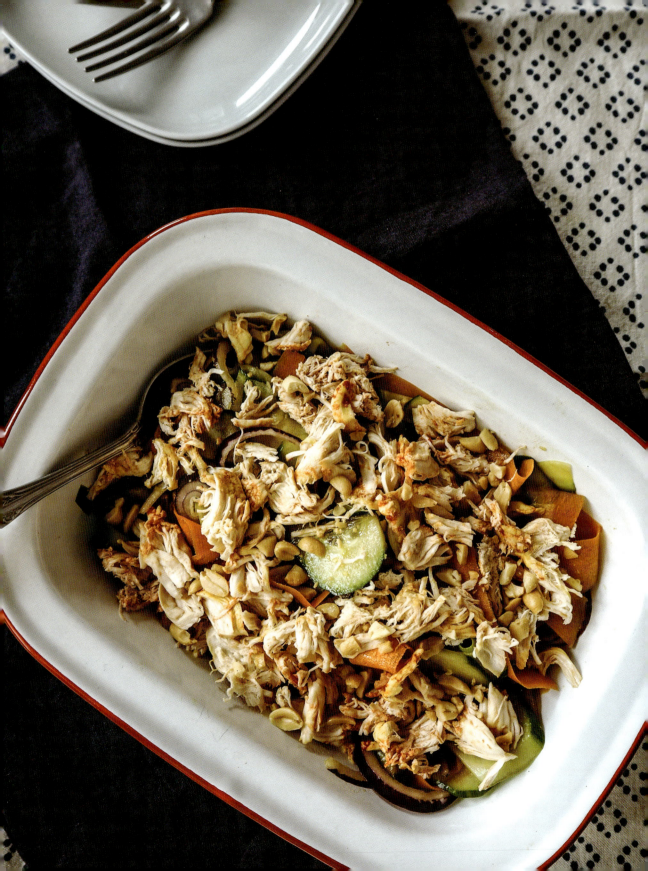

Warm shredded chicken and chilli salad

🍽 **Serves:** 2 ⏱ **Prep time:** 10 mins 🍲 **Cooking time:** 45–50 mins

Ingredients

- 1 tin of coconut milk (low-fat)
- 1 stalk of lemongrass
- 300g/10½oz chicken breast
- 2 tsp. Thai red curry paste
- Fresh coriander
- 100g/3½oz carrot, peeled
- 100g/3½oz courgette
- 100g/3½oz cucumber
- 1 small red onion, peeled
- 20g/³/₄oz peanuts, crushed

Chilli dressing:
- 2 tbsp. rice vinegar
- 2 tbsp. sweet chilli sauce
- 1 tsp. sesame oil
- ¼ tsp. sugar/sweetener

Method

1. Preheat oven to 160°C/320°F (fan 140°C/280°F) or gas mark 3.

2. In an ovenproof dish, pour in the coconut milk and add the lemongrass (chopped).

3. Coat the chicken in the curry paste and add to the dish. Cover and place in the oven until cooked through.

4. While the chicken is cooking, thinly slice the carrot, courgette, cucumber and onion.

5. Make the dressing by mixing the ingredients together.

6. Toss the salad with the dressing.

7. When the chicken is cooked, shred with 2 forks in the reduced coconut milk. Stir through chopped fresh coriander.

8. Top the salad with the poached chicken and sprinkle crushed peanuts on top.

NUTRITION INFORMATION
Amount per serving

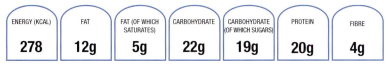

ENERGY (KCAL)	FAT	FAT (OF WHICH SATURATES)	CARBOHYDRATE	CARBOHYDRATE (OF WHICH SUGARS)	PROTEIN	FIBRE
278	12g	5g	22g	19g	20g	4g

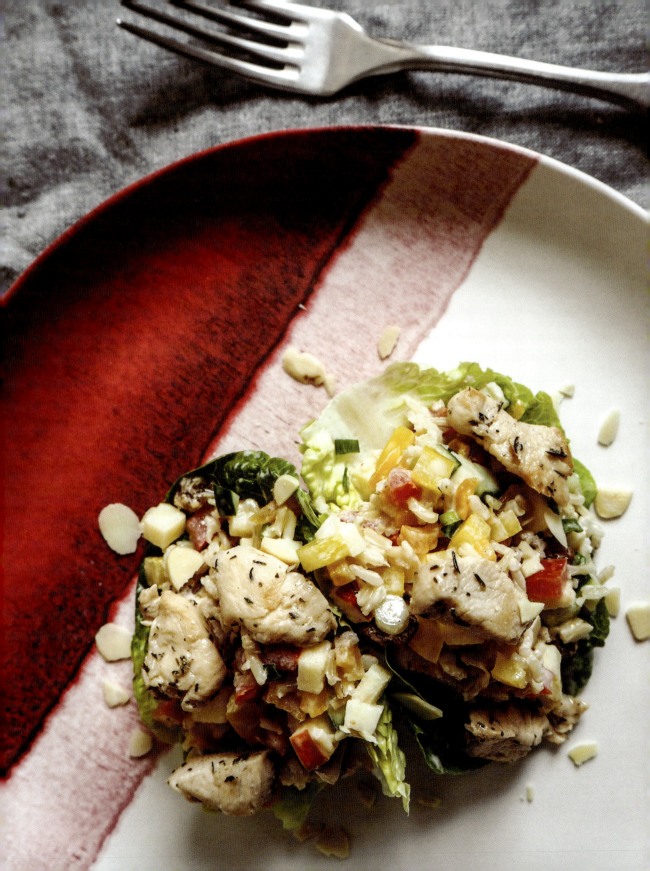

Rainbow salad

🍽 **Serves:** 2 ⏱ **Prep time:** 15 mins

Ingredients

- 1 small gem lettuce
- 8 tbsp. cold pre-cooked brown rice (60g uncooked weight)
- 150g/5oz cold cooked chicken, cut into bite-sized pieces
- 2 medium tomatoes, diced
- 5cm/2in piece of cucumber, diced
- 2 spring onions, finely chopped
- 1 small yellow pepper, diced
- 1 ring pineapple canned in natural juice, drained and cut into small pieces
- ½ red apple, diced (use lemon juice to prevent it turning brown)
- 4 dried apricots, finely chopped
- ½ tbsp. sultanas
- 1 tbsp. flaked almonds

For the vinaigrette:
- 1 tsp. olive oil
- 2 tsp. white wine vinegar
- Freshly ground black pepper
- 1 tbsp. low-fat Greek yogurt

Method

1. Arrange the lettuce leaves on serving plates to look like petals.

2. Place the rice and chicken in a mixing bowl with the remaining ingredients and stir gently together.

3. Make the vinaigrette by mixing the ingredients together. Dress the salad with the vinaigrette and toss lightly. Spoon the salad on to the prepared serving plates on top of the lettuce leaves.

NUTRITION INFORMATION
Amount per serving

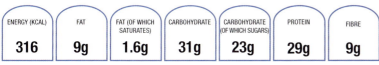

ENERGY (KCAL)	FAT	FAT (OF WHICH SATURATES)	CARBOHYDRATE	CARBOHYDRATE (OF WHICH SUGARS)	PROTEIN	FIBRE
316	9g	1.6g	31g	23g	29g	9g

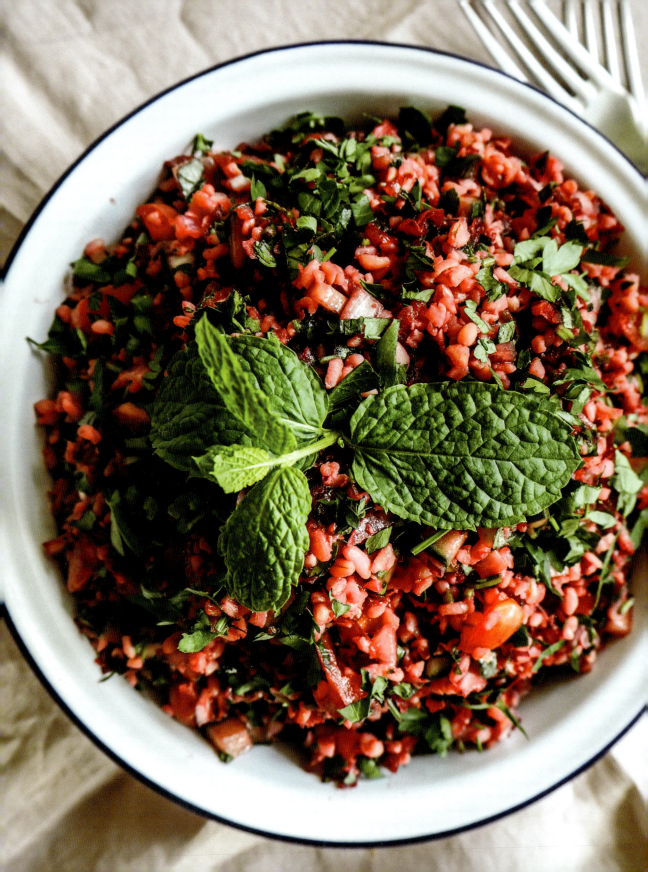

Pink tabbouleh salad

🍽 **Serves:** 4 ⏱ **Prep time:** 30 mins 🍲 **Cooking time:** 30 mins

Ingredients

- ¾ cup/190ml boiling water
- ½ cup/4oz/110g bulgar wheat
- 1 small clove garlic, peeled and minced
- Juice of 1 lemon
- 2 tbsp. olive or rapeseed oil
- Pinch of black pepper
- 1 cucumber, peeled, deseeded and diced
- 4 medium tomatoes, diced
- 4 scallions, finely chopped
- 1 cooked, medium-sized beetroot, peeled and diced
- 4 tbsp. freshly chopped parsley
- 4 tbsp. freshly chopped mint

Method

1. Pour the water over the bulgar wheat. Cover and allow to soak for 30 minutes.

2. Mix the garlic, lemon juice, olive oil and black pepper in a bowl.

3. Remove the cover from the bulgar and fluff the grains with a fork to separate them. This helps them from clumping together. Pour the lemon dressing over the cooked bulgar wheat and stir well. Allow to cool.

4. When the bulgar wheat is cool, mix in the chopped vegetables and herbs.

5. Taste the salad and adjust the seasoning to your liking with additional lemon juice, pepper and herbs.

NUTRITION INFORMATION
Amount per serving

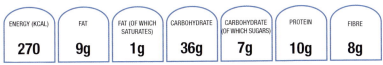

ENERGY (KCAL)	FAT	FAT (OF WHICH SATURATES)	CARBOHYDRATE	CARBOHYDRATE (OF WHICH SUGARS)	PROTEIN	FIBRE
270	9g	1g	36g	7g	10g	8g

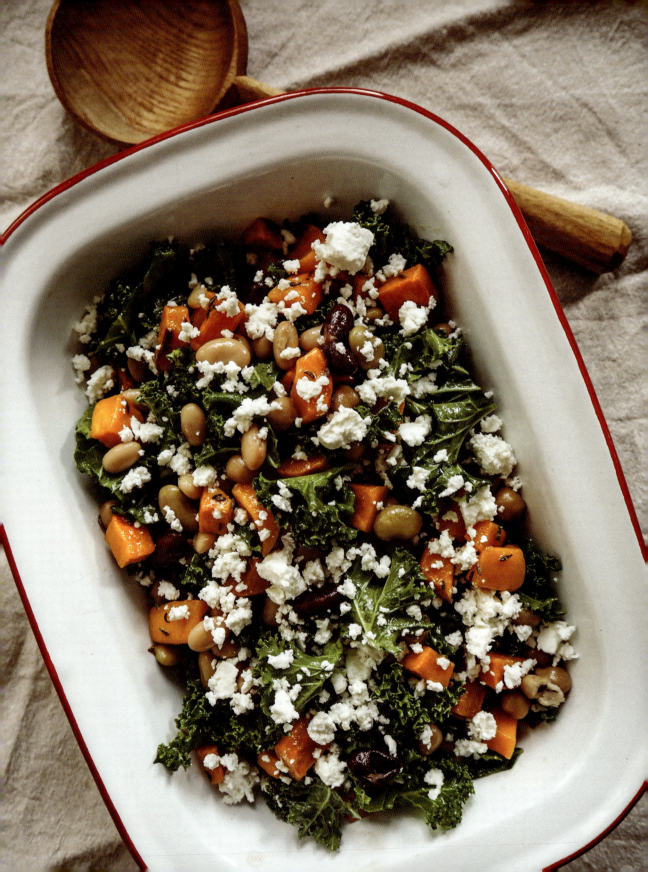

Roast squash, bean and kale salad

Serves: 4 Prep time: 15 mins Cooking time: 30 mins

Ingredients

- 1 butternut squash, peeled and diced
- 1 red onion, peeled and roughly chopped
- 1 tsp. cumin seeds
- ½ tbsp. rapeseed/olive oil
- 1 tin beans, drained – e.g. mixed beans, chickpeas, kidney beans, pinto beans
- 3 leaves kale, de-stalked and finely chopped
- 1 handful freshly chopped parsley
- 75g/3oz feta
- 1 tsp. cracked black pepper

Dressing:
- 1 tsp. Dijon mustard
- 1 tsp. honey
- 1 tbsp. cider vinegar
- 2 tbsp. olive oil

Method

1. Heat the oven to 170°C/325°F (fan 150°C/300°F) or gas mark 3. Place the chopped squash and onion on a flat baking tray. Toss in the cumin seeds and oil, mix to coat. Place in the oven for 30 minutes, turning once halfway through. The squash and onion should both be soft.

2. Meanwhile heat a pan of water until boiling. Add the chopped kale and cook for 30 seconds. Remove with a slotted spoon or drain in a colander and transfer directly to a large serving bowl.

3. Add the beans, half the parsley and the cooked squash/onion to the kale.

4. Make the dressing by combining all the ingredients in a jar and shake well.

5. Pour the dressing over the vegetables and mix to combine.

6. Top the salad with crumbled feta, black pepper and the remaining chopped parsley.

NUTRITION INFORMATION
Amount per serving

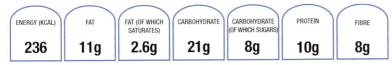

ENERGY (KCAL)	FAT	FAT (OF WHICH SATURATES)	CARBOHYDRATE	CARBOHYDRATE (OF WHICH SUGARS)	PROTEIN	FIBRE
236	11g	2.6g	21g	8g	10g	8g

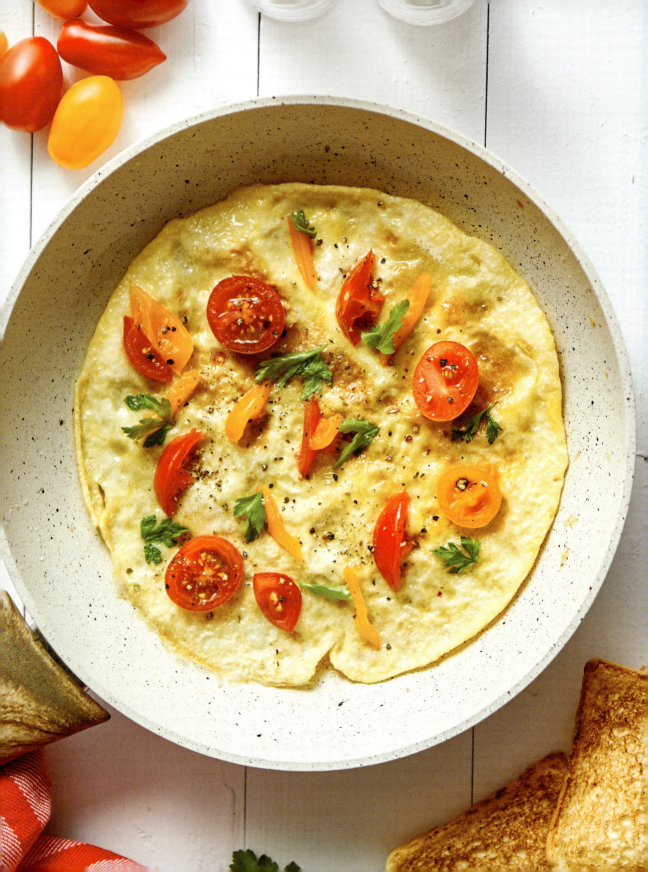

Hot light meals

Chicken fajita stuffed peppers

Courgette and feta fritters

Ranch-style eggs

Spinach and sweet potato tortilla

Mexican beans on toast

Tuna and sweetcorn fritters

Baked potatoes:

- With bean chilli

- With beef chilli

- With chicken, onion and cheese

- With salmon

- With tuna and sweetcorn

- With baked beans

Healthy omelette

Tortilla pizza

Farmers market scramble

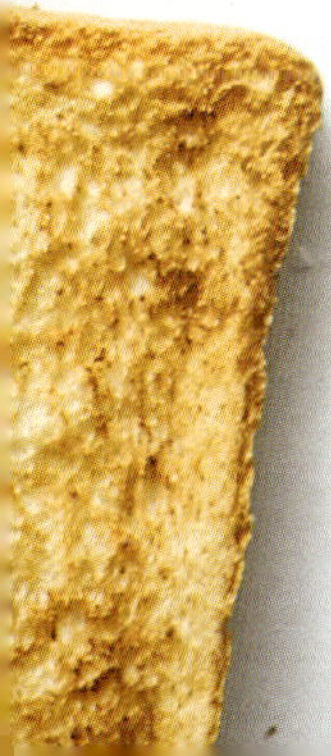

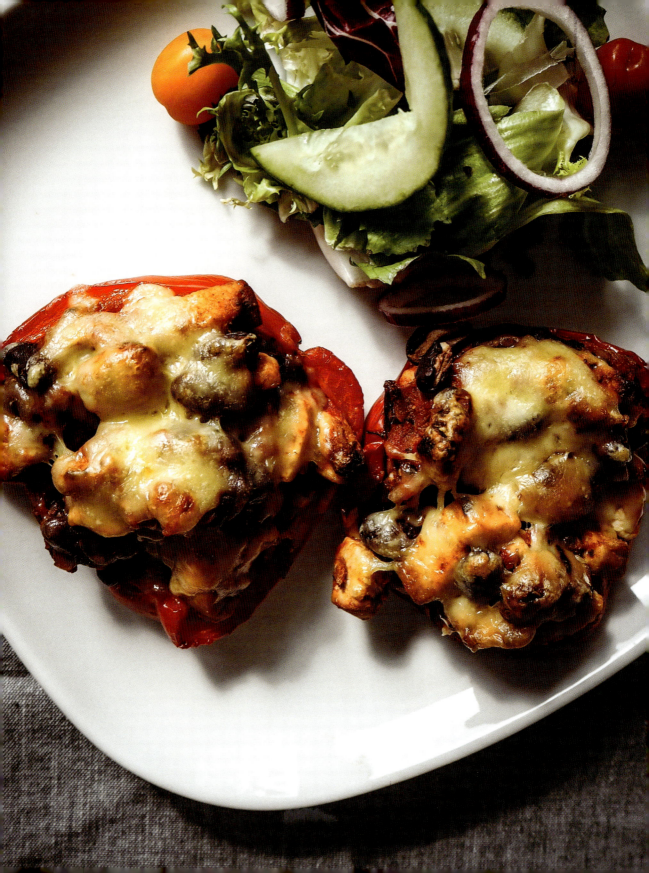

Chicken fajita stuffed peppers

🍽 **Serves:** 6 ⏱ **Prep time:** 10 mins 🍵 **Cooking time:** 1 hour

Ingredients

- 6 red peppers
- 350ml/1½ cups chicken stock
- 1½ tbsp. olive oil
- 1 medium onion, diced
- 3 cloves garlic (minced)
- 3 chicken breasts, cut into chunks
- 1 tbsp. chilli powder
- 1 tsp. ground cumin
- 1 tsp. garlic powder
- 1 tsp. paprika
- 1 x 400g/14oz tin chopped tomatoes
- 1 x 400g/14oz tin red kidney beans
- 60g/½ cup grated low-fat cheddar cheese

Serve with a large side salad.

Method

1. Preheat the oven to 200°C/400°F (fan 180°C/350°F) or gas mark 6.

2. Slice the red peppers in half (lengthways), remove seeds and stems.

3. Pour ⅓ of the chicken stock (115ml/½ cup) into the dish which will be used to roast the peppers in the oven.

4. In a large pan, heat the olive oil. Add the onion and cook for 5 minutes on a low heat, until softened and golden. Add the garlic and stir until fragrant.

5. Add the chicken and seasonings. Cook the chicken, stirring until slightly browned.

6. Add the tomatoes and the remainder of the chicken stock. Bring to the boil, and then allow to simmer for 15 minutes, or until thick, stirring occasionally.

7. Next, mix in the beans and allow to cook for a few more minutes.

8. Spoon the mixture into each pepper half. Cover with foil and bake for 30–35 minutes.

9. Remove the foil from the baking dish, sprinkle each pepper with grated cheese, and place the dish back in the oven to melt the cheese (about 3 minutes).

10. Serve with a large mixed side salad.

NUTRITION INFORMATION
Amount per serving

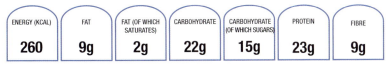

ENERGY (KCAL)	FAT	FAT (OF WHICH SATURATES)	CARBOHYDRATE	CARBOHYDRATE (OF WHICH SUGARS)	PROTEIN	FIBRE
260	9g	2g	22g	15g	23g	9g

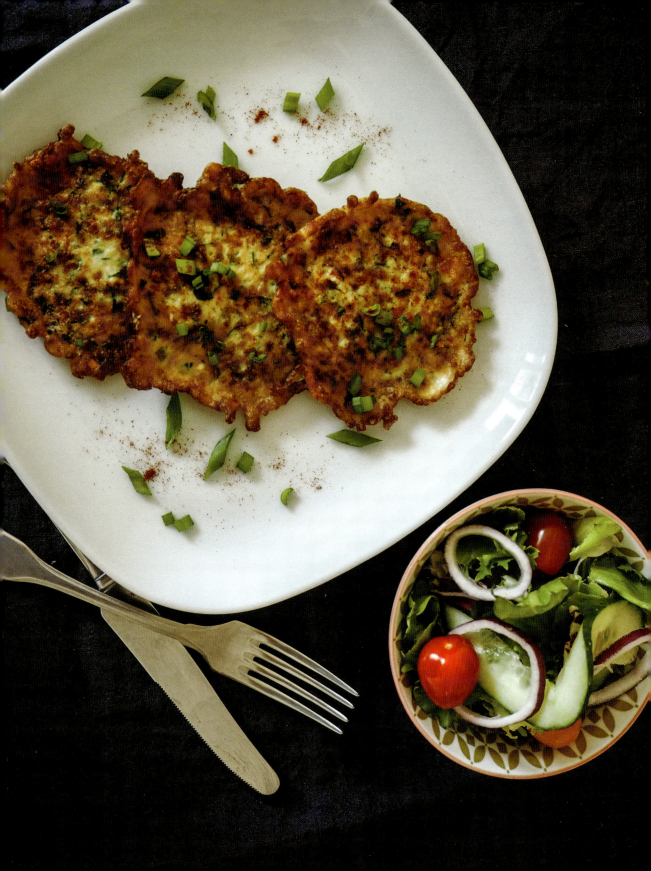

Courgette and feta fritters

Serves: 4 (makes 10–12 fritters) ⏱ Prep time: 10 mins 🍲 Cooking time: 20 mins

Ingredients

- 225g/8oz courgette, grated
- 2 eggs, beaten
- 2 spring onions, finely chopped
- 4 tbsp. plain flour
- 150g/5oz feta, crumbled
- 1 tsp. fresh mint, finely chopped
- Small pinch of chilli flakes
- 2 tbsp. vegetable oil
- Serve with a large side salad

Method

1. Squeeze excess moisture out of the grated courgette.

2. In a bowl, combine the courgette, eggs, onion, flour, feta, mint and chilli. Make sure the ingredients are thoroughly mixed.

3. Heat a small amount of oil in a frying pan over a medium-high heat. Drop a heaped tbsp. of courgette mixture into the pan and cook for 5 minutes on each side until golden.

NUTRITION INFORMATION
Amount per serving

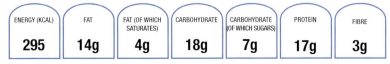

ENERGY (KCAL)	FAT	FAT (OF WHICH SATURATES)	CARBOHYDRATE	CARBOHYDRATE (OF WHICH SUGARS)	PROTEIN	FIBRE
295	14g	4g	18g	7g	17g	3g

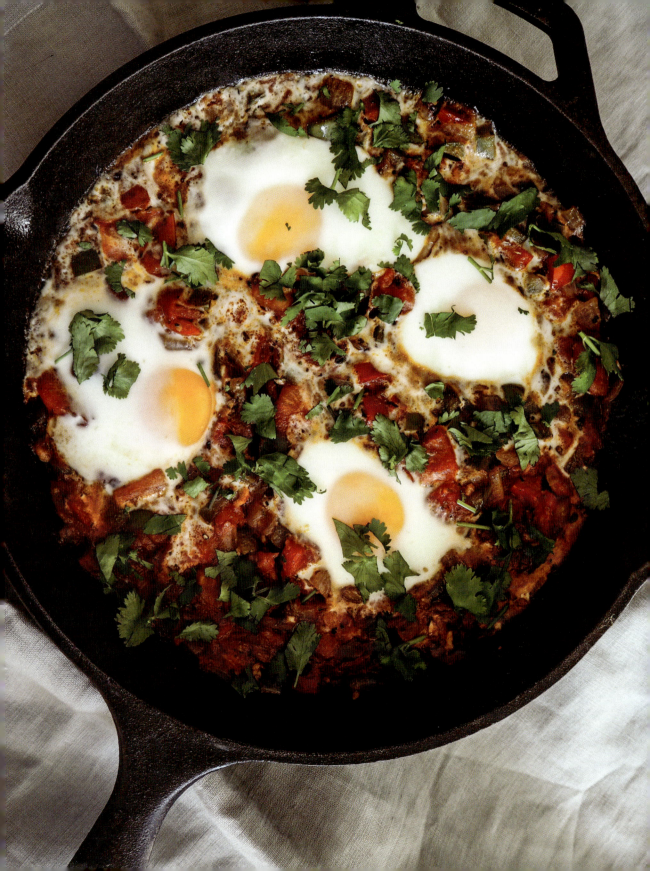

Ranch-style eggs

🍽 **Serves:** 2 ⏱ **Prep time:** 5 mins 🍲 **Cooking time:** 20 mins

Ingredients

- 1 tbsp. olive oil
- 1 small onion, thinly sliced
- 1 red chilli, deseeded and finely chopped
- 1 garlic clove, crushed
- 1 tsp. cumin
- 1 tsp. paprika
- 1 tsp. oregano
- 1 green pepper, diced
- 1 red pepper, diced
- 1 x 400g/14oz tin of tomatoes
- Freshly ground black pepper
- 4 eggs
- Fresh chopped coriander to garnish

Method

1. Heat the oil in a large frying pan and add the onion. Cook for 5 minutes then add the chilli, garlic, cumin, paprika, oregano and peppers.

2. Fry for about 3 minutes then add the tomatoes. Bring to the boil and cook for another 5 minutes.

3. Season with pepper and then make 4 hollows in the mixture. Break an egg into each and cover the pan with a lid. Cook for 3–5 minutes or until the eggs are just set.

4. Serve immediately, garnished with chopped coriander.

NUTRITION INFORMATION
Amount per serving

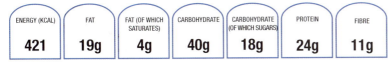

ENERGY (KCAL)	FAT	FAT (OF WHICH SATURATES)	CARBOHYDRATE	CARBOHYDRATE (OF WHICH SUGARS)	PROTEIN	FIBRE
421	19g	4g	40g	18g	24g	11g

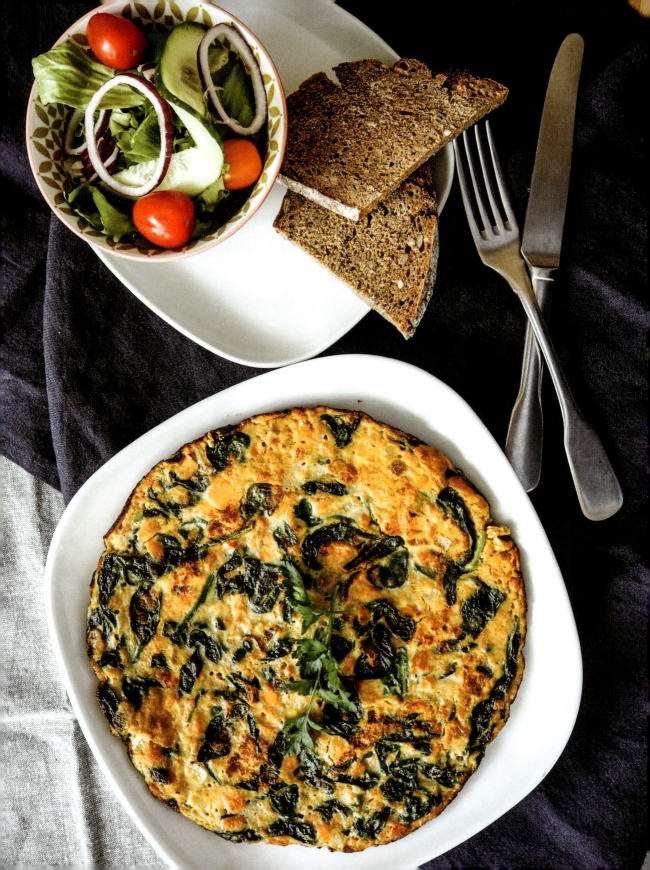

Spinach and sweet potato tortilla

🍽️ **Serves:** 4 ⏱️ **Prep time:** 10 mins 🍵 **Cooking time:** 1 hour

Ingredients

- 150g/¾ cup baby spinach
- 2 tbsp. olive oil
- 1 large onion, peeled and thinly sliced
- Freshly ground black pepper
- 400g/14oz sweet potato, peeled and thinly sliced
- 1 garlic clove, finely chopped
- 4 eggs

Serve with brown bread/toast and a large side salad.

Method

1. Put the spinach in a large colander and pour over a kettleful of boiling water. Drain well and, when cooled a little, squeeze dry.

2. Heat 1 tbsp. oil in a non-stick pan with a lid. Sweat the onions for 10 minutes until really soft but not coloured.

3. Mix the potatoes and garlic in with the onions, season well, cover and cook over a gentle heat, stirring occasionally, for another 15 minutes until the potatoes are tender.

4. Whisk the eggs in a large bowl, tip in the cooked potato and onion, and mix together. Separate the spinach clumps, add to the mix and fold through, trying not to break up the potato too much.

5. Add 1 tbsp of oil to the pan and add the sweet potato and egg mixture. Cover with a lid and cook over a low-medium heat for 20 minutes until the base and sides are golden brown and the centre has mostly set.

6. Run a palette knife around the sides to stop it from sticking. To turn the tortilla over, put a plate face down onto the pan, then flip it over. Slide the tortilla back into the pan and cook for a further 5–10 minutes until just set and golden all over. Alternatively, instead of flipping the tortilla over you may finish it under the grill for 5 minutes.

7. Serve with a slice of fresh brown bread/toast and a side salad.

NUTRITION INFORMATION
Amount per serving

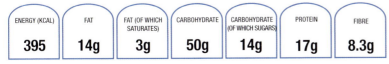

ENERGY (KCAL)	FAT	FAT (OF WHICH SATURATES)	CARBOHYDRATE	CARBOHYDRATE (OF WHICH SUGARS)	PROTEIN	FIBRE
395	14g	3g	50g	14g	17g	8.3g

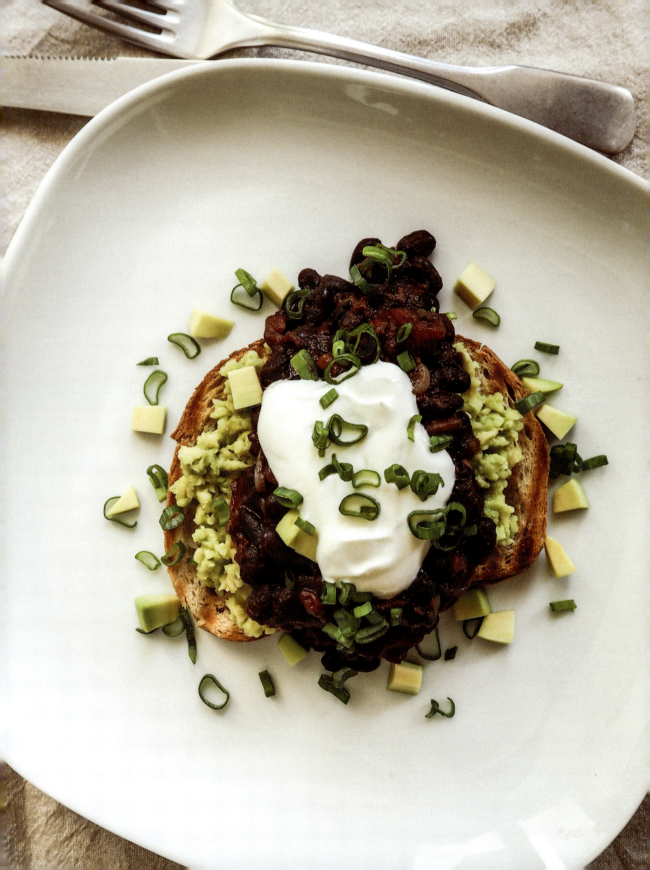

Mexican beans on toast

Serves: 2 **Prep time:** 5 mins **Cooking time:** 15 minutes

Ingredients

- 1 x 400g/14oz tin chopped tomatoes
- 2 spring onions, whites and greens separated, both finely sliced
- 2 tsp. ground cumin
- 2 tsp. mild chilli powder
- 1 tbsp. brown or barbecue sauce
- 1 x 400g/14oz tin black beans
- 2 slices of wholemeal bread
- 1 small ripe avocado
- A few good squeezes of lemon or lime juice
- 2 tbsp. natural yogurt

Method

1. Add the tomatoes, onion whites, spices and brown/barbecue sauce into a saucepan. Bring to a simmer and allow to bubble for 10 minutes.

2. Stir in the beans and heat through for 5 minutes. Meanwhile, toast the bread, then dice half the avocado and mix with a few squeezes of lemon or lime juice.

3. Mash the remaining half avocado on the toast. Top with the hot beans followed by the diced avocado and yogurt. Scatter with the spring onion greens to garnish.

NUTRITION INFORMATION
Amount per serving

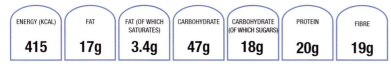

ENERGY (KCAL)	FAT	FAT (OF WHICH SATURATES)	CARBOHYDRATE	CARBOHYDRATE (OF WHICH SUGARS)	PROTEIN	FIBRE
415	17g	3.4g	47g	18g	20g	19g

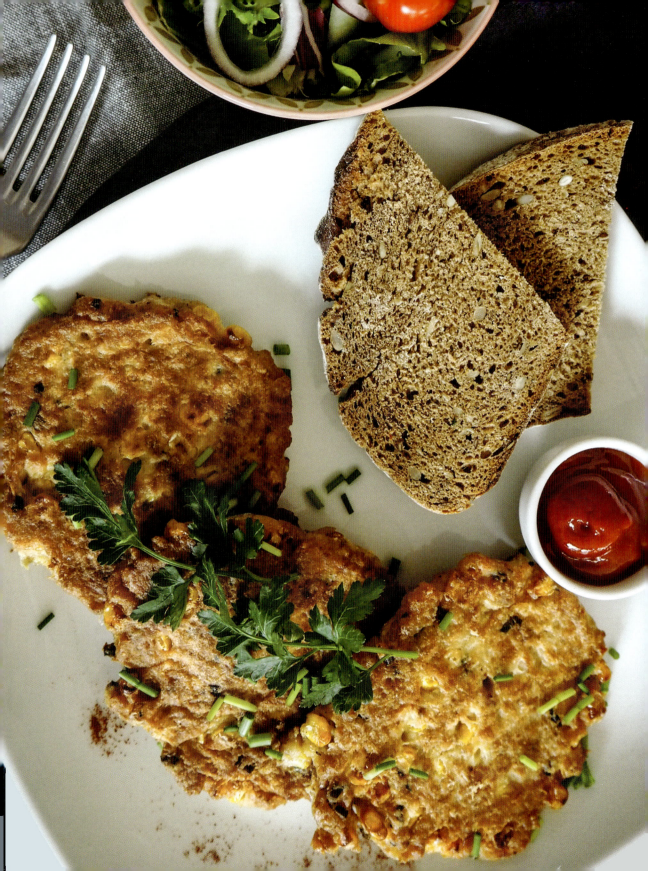

Tuna and sweetcorn fritters

Serves: 4 (makes 8 fritters) **Prep time:** 5 mins **Cooking time:** 15 minutes

Ingredients

- 2 x 120g/4oz tins tuna, drained
- 1 x 140g/5oz tin sweetcorn
- 2 tbsp. plain flour
- 1 egg yolk
- 1 spring onion, thinly sliced
- 1 tbsp. olive oil or rapeseed oil
- Large mixed salad to serve and a slice of brown bread
- Chilli sauce to serve

Method

1. Flake the tuna into a bowl, drain the sweetcorn and mix the two together.

2. Add the flour, egg yolk and spring onion, and mix together well.

3. Heat a little oil in a frying pan over a medium heat.

4. When hot, spoon a large tbsp. of the mix into the pan and repeat to make about 8 small fritters.

5. Fry for about 5 minutes on each side until browned and cooked through.

6. Serve with some chilli sauce if desired and a large green salad.

NUTRITION INFORMATION
Amount per serving

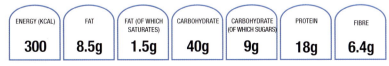

ENERGY (KCAL)	FAT	FAT (OF WHICH SATURATES)	CARBOHYDRATE	CARBOHYDRATE (OF WHICH SUGARS)	PROTEIN	FIBRE
300	8.5g	1.5g	40g	9g	18g	6.4g

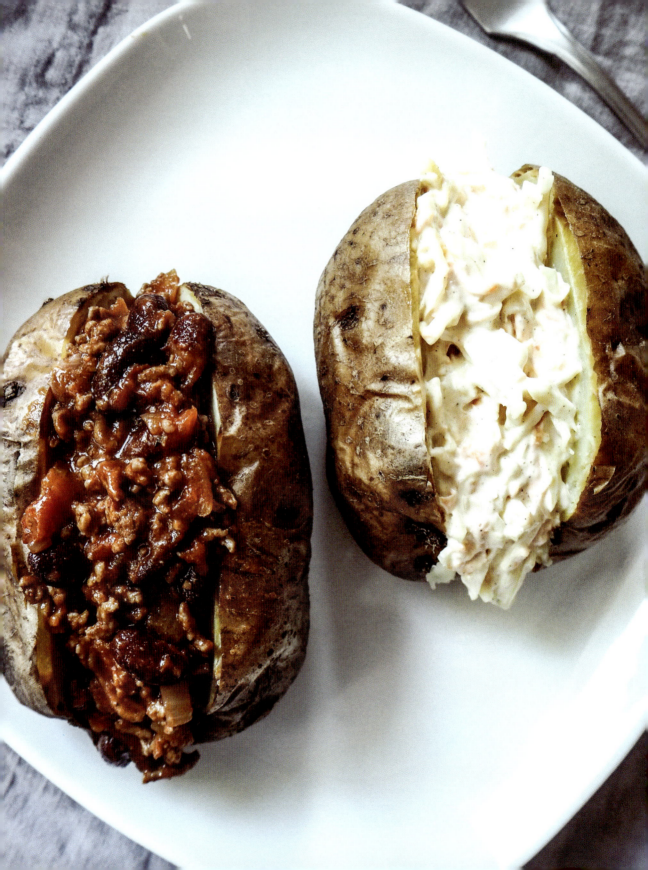

Baked potatoes

🍽 **Serves:** 4 ⏱ **Prep time:** 5–10 mins 🍲 **Cooking time:** ~1 hour

Ingredients

- 4 large baking potatoes, washed and skin left on
- 2 tsp. olive oil

Toppings:
- Flaked cooked/tinned salmon, 1 tbsp. low-fat mayo, 1 tsp. capers and squeeze lemon
- Tinned tuna, 1 tbsp. low-fat mayo, handful tinned sweetcorn (drained)
- Baked beans or mexican beans
- Leftover chilli con carne (see page 185) or bean chilli (see page 265)
- Chunky salsa (see page 173) and grated cheese
- Chicken, spring onions and 1 tbsp. low-fat cream cheese

Method

1. Heat the oven to 220°C/425°F (fan 200°C /400°F) or gas mark 7. Rub a little oil over each potato and bake on the top shelf of the oven for 20 minutes, then turn down the oven to 190°C/375°F (fan 170°C /325°F) or gas mark 5 and bake for 45 minutes–1 hour until the skin is crisp and the flesh soft.

2. Cut a cross in the cooked potato to split it open and top with a topping of your choice. Alternatively scoop out the potato filling, mix with your topping of choice and refill the baked potato.

NUTRITION INFORMATION
Amount per serving

	ENERGY (KCAL)	FAT	FAT (OF WHICH SATURATES)	CARBOHYDRATE	CARBOHYDRATE (OF WHICH SUGARS)	PROTEIN	FIBRE
Bean chilli	370	4g	0.7g	67g	16g	14g	16g
Beef chilli	305	6g	1.4g	46g	6g	13g	8g
Chicken, onion and cheese	320	4g	1.6g	43g	4g	27g	6g
Salmon and capers	340	8g	1.3g	42g	3g	24g	5g
Tuna and sweetcorn	330	5.3g	0.8g	46g	5g	23g	6g
Baked beans	344	1.4g	0.4g	66g	9g	15g	15g
Chunky salsa and grated cheese	340	7.5g	1.3g	60g	6g	7g	8g

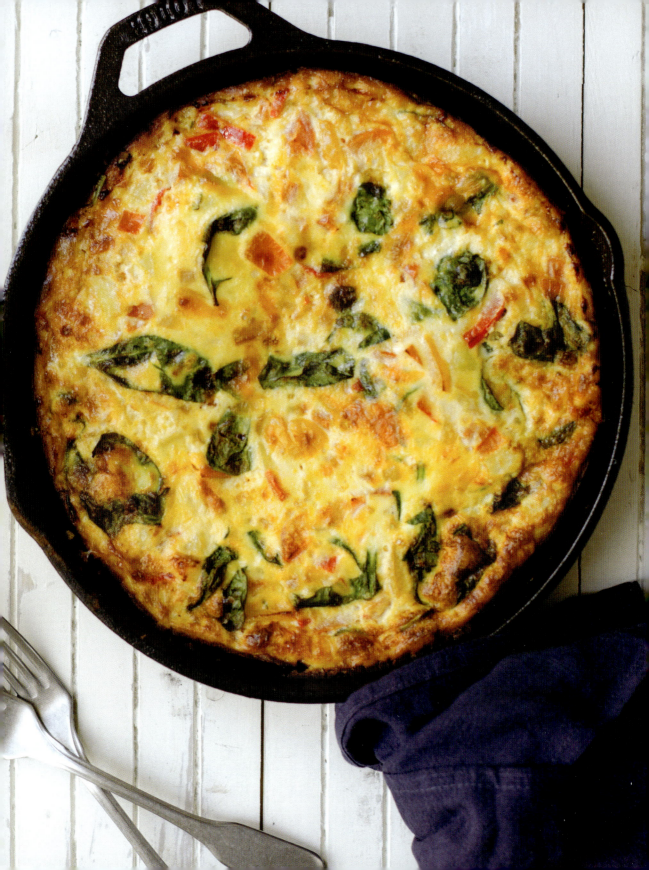

Healthy omelette

🍽 **Serves:** 2 ⏱ **Prep time:** 10 mins 🍲 **Cooking time:** <10 mins

Ingredients

- 2 eggs
- 3 egg whites
- Freshly ground black pepper
- 1 tsp. olive oil or rapeseed oil
- 2 spring onions, chopped
- 2 large tomatoes, chopped
- 80g/1 cup mushrooms, sliced
- 80g/½ cup spinach leaves
- 40g/$\frac{1}{3}$ cup grated low-fat cheddar cheese

Method

1. Whisk the eggs and egg whites together and season with black pepper.

2. Add oil to a large frying pan and heat over a medium-high heat.

3. Add the tomatoes, mushrooms and onions and cook, stirring once or twice, until softened, 1 to 2 minutes. Place the spinach on top, cover and let wilt, about 30 seconds. Stir to combine.

4. Add the egg mixture to the frying pan, covering all of the vegetables. Sprinkle cheese over if desired. Cook over a medium heat until completely set.

NUTRITION INFORMATION
Amount per serving

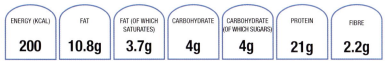

ENERGY (KCAL)	FAT	FAT (OF WHICH SATURATES)	CARBOHYDRATE	CARBOHYDRATE (OF WHICH SUGARS)	PROTEIN	FIBRE
200	10.8g	3.7g	4g	4g	21g	2.2g

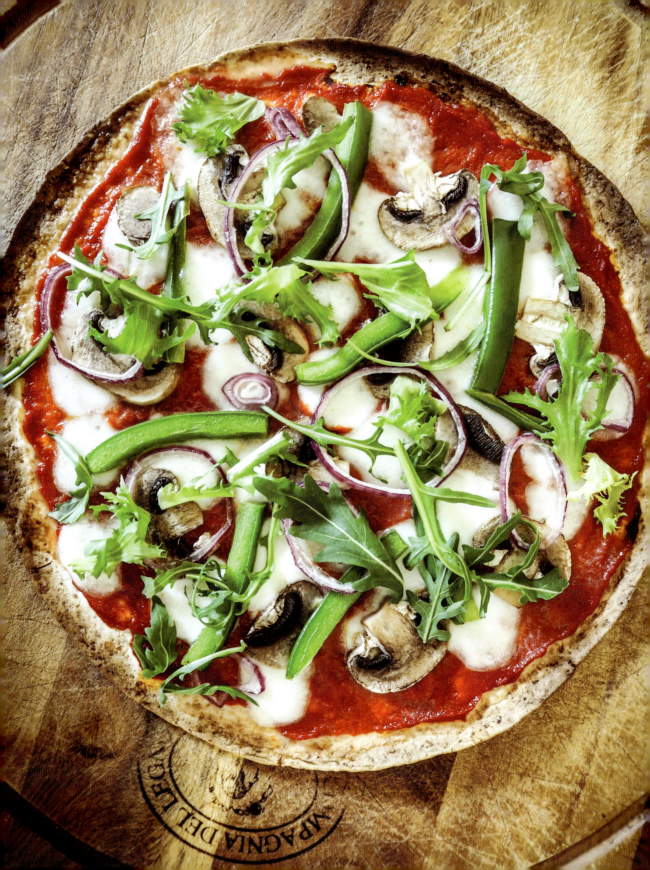

Tortilla pizza

🍽 **Serves:** 4 ⏱ **Prep time:** 5 mins 🍲 **Cooking time:** <10 mins

Ingredients

- Mix 1 tbsp. passata with 1 tsp. tomato puree for each wrap
- 4 wholemeal soft tortilla wraps
- 1 x 125g/4oz ball of reduced-fat mozzarella, drained

Toppings:
- 80g/1 cup mushrooms
- ½ tsp. smoked paprika
- 1 small red onion, finely sliced
- ½ fresh pepper, sliced
- Rocket to garnish pizzas

Serve with a large side salad.

Method

1. Preheat the oven and baking trays to 220°C/425°F (fan 200°C/400°F) or gas mark 7.

2. Place the tortillas on a clean, dry surface. The tortillas will form the base of the pizza. Using the back of a spoon, evenly coat the tortillas with the tomato sauce, leaving a 2cm edge for the crust.

3. Tear the mozzarella into small pieces. Add a quarter to each pizza, spreading the pieces out evenly.

4. Place the sliced mushrooms into a bowl and sprinkle the paprika over the top. Toss gently to coat all slices with the paprika.

5. Add the slices of mushroom, red onion and pepper to all the pizzas.

6. Carefully remove the baking trays from the oven. Transfer the pizzas onto the trays and place them back in the oven. Cook for 3–5 minutes, until the cheese has melted and the crusts are golden.

7. Garnish with rocket and serve with a side salad.

NUTRITION INFORMATION
Amount per serving

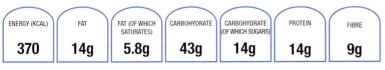

ENERGY (KCAL)	FAT	FAT (OF WHICH SATURATES)	CARBOHYDRATE	CARBOHYDRATE (OF WHICH SUGARS)	PROTEIN	FIBRE
370	14g	5.8g	43g	14g	14g	9g

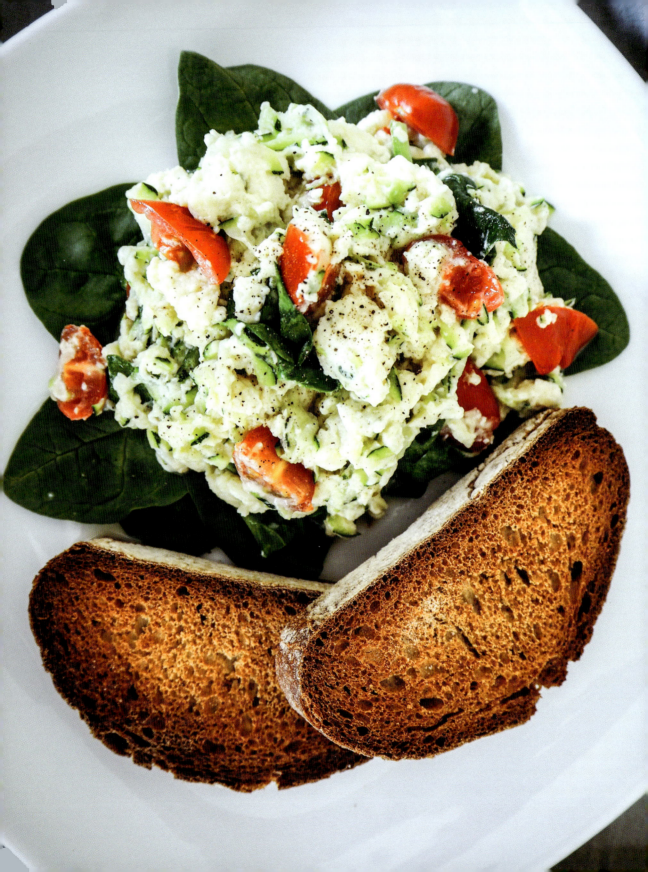

Farmers market scramble

🍽 **Serves:** 4 ⏱ **Prep time:** 5 mins 🍲 **Cooking time:** 6 mins

Ingredients

- 8 large eggs
- 2 tbsp. low-fat milk
- Freshly ground black pepper
- 3 tsp. olive oil
- 1 small courgette (130g/5oz) diced
- 16 cherry tomatoes (120g/$^2/_3$ cup), seeded and diced
- 30g/1oz baby spinach leaves

Method

1. In a bowl whisk together the eggs, milk and a pinch of pepper. Set aside.

2. Warm the oil in non-stick pan over medium heat. Add the courgette and cook until tender (about 2 minutes). Add the tomato and stir to combine.

3. Reduce the heat to medium-low, add the egg mixture and let cook, without stirring, until the eggs just begin to set, about 1 minute. Using a heatproof rubber spatula gently push the eggs around the pan to cook any remaining uncooked egg.

4. When the eggs are half cooked (1–2 minutes longer), add the spinach. Stir gently to combine and continue cooking until the eggs are completely cooked but still moist (another minute).

5. Transfer to a warm plate and serve.

NUTRITION INFORMATION
Amount per serving

ENERGY (KCAL)	FAT	FAT (OF WHICH SATURATES)	CARBOHYDRATE	CARBOHYDRATE (OF WHICH SUGARS)	PROTEIN	FIBRE
218.1	15.3g	4.2g	2.2g	2g	18.1g	1.2g

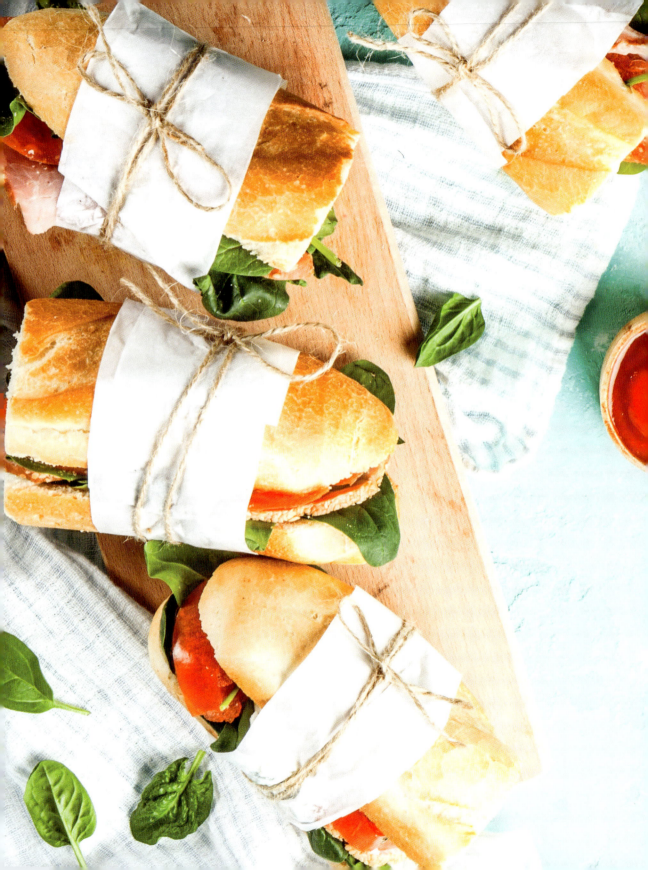

Sandwiches and wraps

Chicken pesto wrap

Spicy chicken pitta

Falafel wraps

Pitta with chicken, carrot and coriander salad

Healthy sandwich fillings

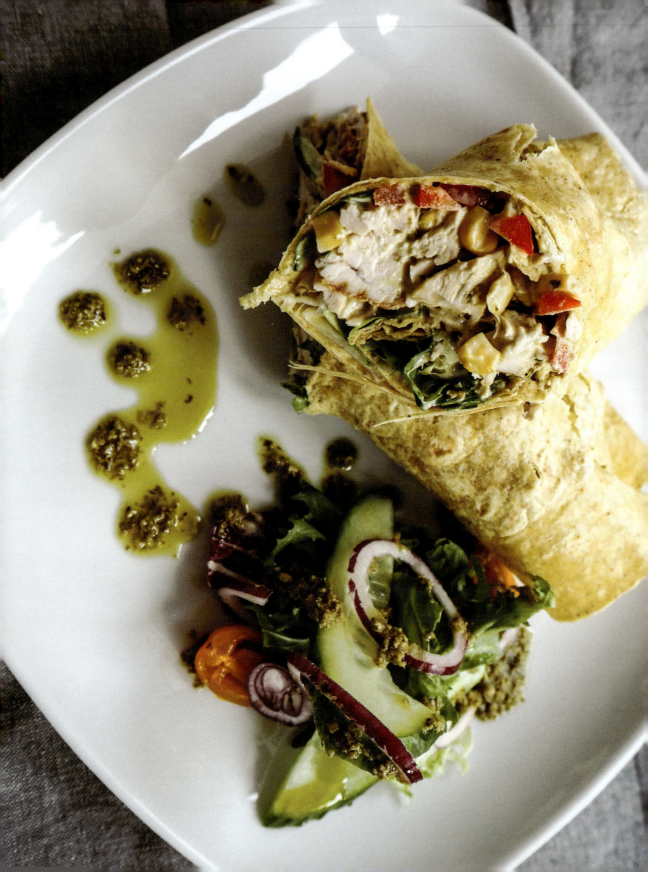

Chicken pesto wrap

🍽 **Serves:** 2 ⏱ **Prep time:** 10 mins

Ingredients

- 1 small chicken breast, boiled/grilled without skin, shredded
- 2 wholemeal tortilla wraps
- 2 tbsp. of low-fat mayonnaise
- 1 tsp. pesto
- Freshly ground black pepper
- ½ large red pepper, sliced
- 1 small tin of sweetcorn, drained
- 60g/2½oz lettuce
- 60g/½ cup cucumber, sliced in strips

Method

1. Mix together the shredded chicken, low-fat mayonnaise and pesto. Season with pepper.

2. Divide the chicken mixture between the wraps. Top with the red pepper, sweetcorn, cucumber and lettuce leaves.

NUTRITION INFORMATION
Amount per serving

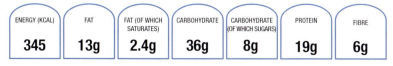

ENERGY (KCAL)	FAT	FAT (OF WHICH SATURATES)	CARBOHYDRATE	CARBOHYDRATE (OF WHICH SUGARS)	PROTEIN	FIBRE
345	13g	2.4g	36g	8g	19g	6g

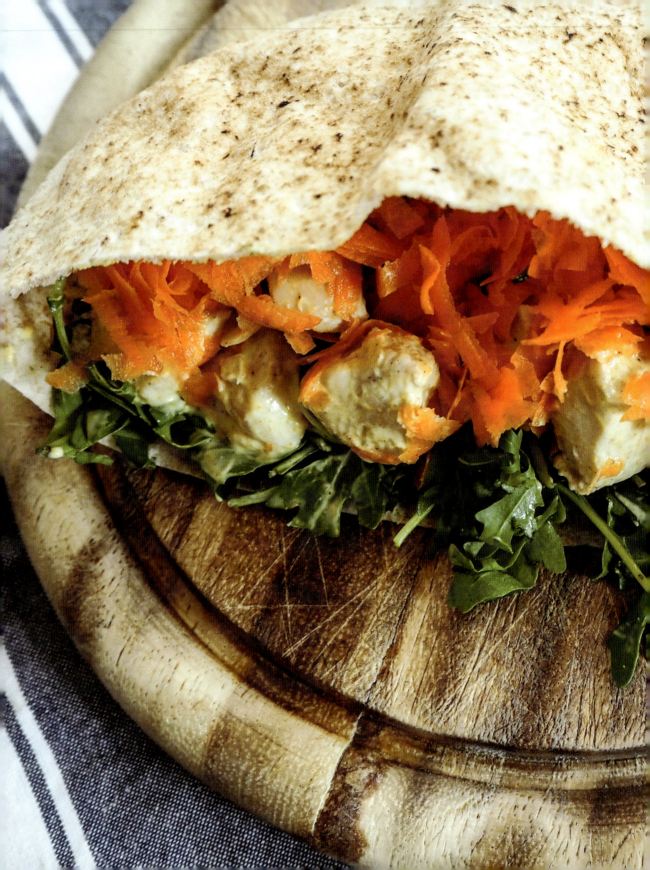

Spicy chicken pitta

Serves: 1 **Prep time:** 10 mins **Cooking time:** 5–10 mins

Ingredients

- 1 tsp. olive oil
- 1 chicken breast, diced, skinless
- 2 tbsp. flaked almonds
- 2 tbsp. natural, low-fat yogurt
- ½ tsp. curry powder
- ¼ tsp. cinnamon
- ¼ tsp. turmeric
- 1 wholemeal pitta
- 1 carrot, peeled and grated
- Small handful rocket leaves

Method

1. Heat the oil in a pan and cook the chicken for about 5 minutes, until golden and cooked through. Set aside to cool.

2. Mix the almonds, yogurt, curry powder, cinnamon and turmeric in a small bowl. Add the cooked chicken and stir well.

3. Quickly toast the pitta on both sides.

4. Split open the pitta and stuff with the chicken mixture, carrot and rocket.

5. Serve immediately.

NUTRITION INFORMATION
Amount per serving

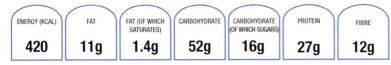

ENERGY (KCAL)	FAT	FAT (OF WHICH SATURATES)	CARBOHYDRATE	CARBOHYDRATE (OF WHICH SUGARS)	PROTEIN	FIBRE
420	11g	1.4g	52g	16g	27g	12g

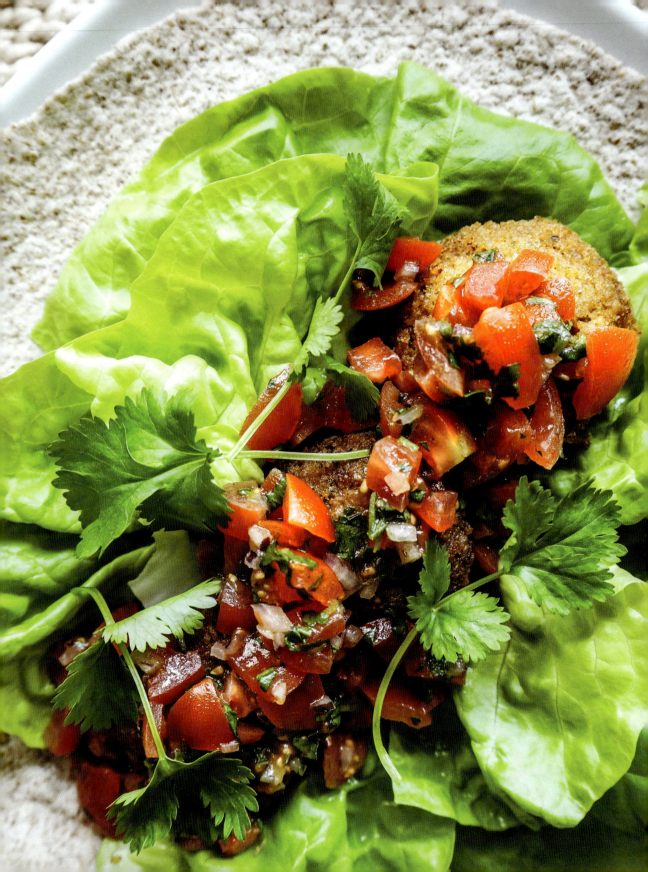

Falafel wraps

🍽 **Serves:** 4 ⏱ **Prep time:** 15 mins 🍲 **Cooking time:** 10 mins

Ingredients

- 1 x 400g/14oz tin of mixed beans
- 1 x 400g/14oz tin of chickpeas
- Zest of 1 lemon
- Pinch of freshly ground black pepper
- 1½ tbsp. harissa paste
- 1 heaped tsp. ground cumin
- 1 heaped tsp. ground coriander
- 1 heaped tbsp. plain flour
- 1 bunch of fresh coriander
- Olive oil
- 4 wholemeal wraps (4 x small 40g/1½oz wraps)
- Green salad (100g/3½oz)
- Salsa (see page 173)

Method

1. Drain the beans and chickpeas and put them into a food processor.

2. Add the finely grated lemon zest, pinch of black pepper, harissa paste, spices, flour and coriander stalks (retain the leaves). Blend to a smooth consistency.

3. Scrape out the mixture and divide and shape into 8 burgers about 1.5cm/½in thick using wet hands.

4. Put 1 tbsp of oil into the frying pan and add the falafels, turning when golden and crisp.

5. Heat the wraps in a microwave.

6. Serve the falafel with lots of green salad and salsa in a warm wholemeal wrap.

NUTRITION INFORMATION
Amount per serving

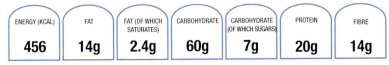

ENERGY (KCAL)	FAT	FAT (OF WHICH SATURATES)	CARBOHYDRATE	CARBOHYDRATE (OF WHICH SUGARS)	PROTEIN	FIBRE
456	14g	2.4g	60g	7g	20g	14g

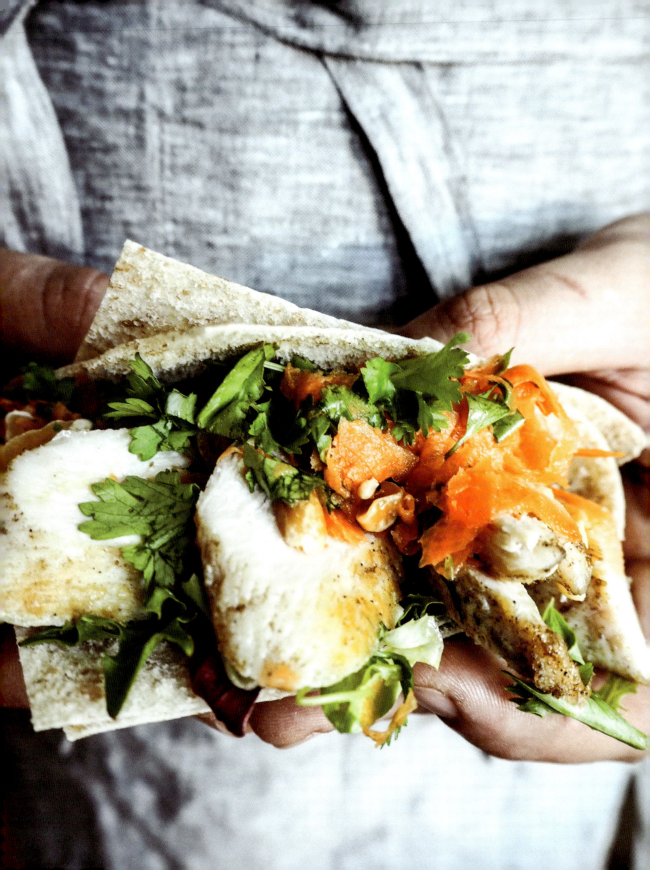

Pitta with chicken, carrot and coriander salad

🍽 Serves: 4 **⏱ Prep time:** 15 mins

Ingredients

- 2 tsp. sugar
- Juice of a lemon or 2 limes
- 4–5 large carrots, peeled and grated
- Small handful of roasted peanuts/Brazil nuts
- 1–2 tbsp. fresh coriander leaves, chopped
- Pinch of black pepper
- 4 wholemeal brown pittas
- 2 chicken breasts, grilled and sliced
- Mixed salad leaves

Method

1. Mix the sugar and lemon juice until all the sugar has dissolved.

2. Put the grated carrot, peanuts and coriander in a large bowl and season to taste with pepper. Pour over the dressing and toss well.

3. Fill a brown pitta with the carrot salad, sliced chicken and mixed green salad leaves.

NUTRITION INFORMATION
Amount per serving

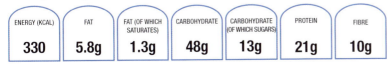

ENERGY (KCAL)	FAT	FAT (OF WHICH SATURATES)	CARBOHYDRATE	CARBOHYDRATE (OF WHICH SUGARS)	PROTEIN	FIBRE
330	5.8g	1.3g	48g	13g	21g	10g

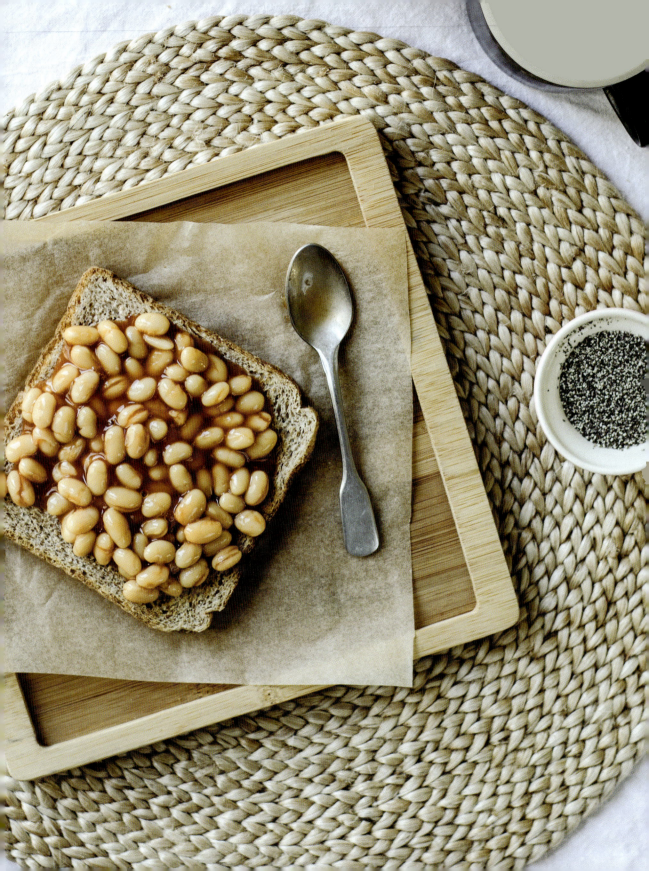

Healthy sandwich fillings: pick & mix

Everyone has their own favourite sandwiches but below we have listed various types of breads, spreads and fillings that will allow you to build your own sandwich and be aware of the nutritional composition.

Examples of breads	Portion control (1 portion should = 125-175 kcal)	Average calories per portion
Brown bread/soda bread	2 small/1½ medium slices	158/175
Wholemeal/wholegrain loaf	2 thin slices	180
Wholemeal wrap	1 small wrap/1 medium wrap	124/170
Brown roll	1 medium roll or ½ large roll	150/100
Brown pitta	1 oval pitta	174
Wholemeal bagel	¾ large bagel or 1 bagel 'slim'	162/120
Rye crispbreads	4 pieces	136
Brown scone	1 small scone	132

Examples of spreads	Portion control	Average calories per portion
Butter	1 tsp.	67
Low-fat spread	1 tsp.	36
Low-fat/'lighter than light' mayonnaise	1 tbsp.	63/15
Low-fat cream cheese spread	1 tbsp.	78
Cottage cheese	1 tbsp.	41
Hummus/reduced-fat hummus	1 tbsp.	89/62
Tomato ketchup (reduced sugar and salt)	1 tbsp.	14
Relish	1 tbsp.	71
Chutney	1 tbsp.	41
Salsa	1 tbsp.	27
Pesto	1 tsp.	34
Mashed avocado	1 tbsp.	57
Peanut butter (no added salt)	1 tsp.	47
Marmalade (no added sugar)	1 tbsp.	45
Jam (no added sugar)	1 tbsp.	45

Examples of meat/fish/alternatives	Portion Control = 2 servings per day 1 serving shown below	Average calories per portion (for example given)
Poultry, e.g. grilled chicken	50–75g/2–3oz cooked	158/175
Fish, tinned/cold fish, e.g. tinned tuna	100g/3½oz	99
Cooked soy/tofu, e.g. steamed tofu	100g/3½oz	73
Egg, e.g. hardboiled	2 eggs	144
Low-fat cheese, e.g. cheddar	Matchbox size (only choose cheese max. once a day)	93
Beans or lentils, e.g. baked beans (no added sugar)	¾ cup	70

Bulk your sandwich up with lots of vegetables/fruit

Examples:

- Apple
- Beetroot
- Celery
- Cucumber
- Grated cabbage
- Grated carrot
- Kale
- Lettuce
- Onion/spring onion
- Peppers
- Pineapple
- Radishes
- Rocket
- Spinach leaves
- Sweetcorn
- Tomato

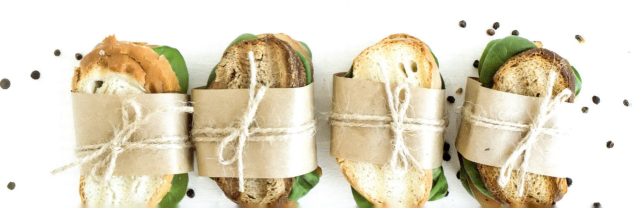

Sandwich ideas

1. **Tuna and sweetcorn:** Low-fat or 'lighter than light' mayonnaise mixed with drained tinned tuna (in spring water) and a handful of sweetcorn.

2. **Egg salad:** Low-fat or 'lighter than light' mayonnaise mixed with mashed/sliced hardboiled eggs and green leaves.

3. **Turkey salad:** Choice of spread with sliced turkey and mixed salad.

4. **Beans on toast:** Toasted wholemeal/wholegrain bread topped with hot baked beans.

5. **Avocado:** Light cream cheese with slices of avocado, cucumber and rocket leaves.

6. **Cheese and onion:** Relish/chutney, low-fat cheese, spring onions, sliced tomatoes and mixed salad leaves.

7. **Creamy salmon:** Drained, tinned salmon mixed with a tsp. capers (rinsed), low-fat mayo/low-fat cream cheese and mixed salad leaves.

8. **Grilled vegetables:** Wholemeal wrap with a tsp. pesto or a tbsp. crumbled feta, an assortment of grilled vegetables (e.g. peppers, courgette and tomatoes) and salad leaves.

9. **Waldorf salad:** Grilled chicken, sliced/grated apple, grapes, celery, low-fat mayonnaise and mixed salad.

10. **Hummus:** Hummus with layers of sliced tomato, cucumber, red onion and spinach leaves.

11. **Curried chicken:** Chicken coated with curry spices and grilled. Slice and mix with low-fat mayo, grated carrot, 1 tsp. currants and mixed leaves.

12. **Greek:** Avocado, tomato, cucumber, red onion, feta, mint and mixed leaves.

13. **Grilled pepper:** Cottage cheese, grilled red peppers and spinach leaves.

14. **Prawn cocktail:** Mix 1 tbsp. of low-fat mayo, 1 tsp. ketchup, 1 drop of Worcestershire sauce and a squeeze of lemon to make a quick marie-rose sauce. Mix with cooked prawns, cucumber, cherry tomatoes and crisp lettuce and serve on brown/soda bread.

15. **Tandoori chicken:** Grilled chicken coated with tandoori spices, cucumber, spinach leaves and a tbsp. low-fat natural yogurt.

16. **Mexican:** Grilled chicken, salsa, sweetcorn, iceberg lettuce, coriander and a squeeze of lime juice.

17. **Roasted veggies and hummus:** Chop a mix of peppers, onions, tomatoes and other favourite veg of choice, then roast with a sprinkle of dried mixed herbs. Once cooked, combine with hummus and spinach in your bread of choice.

18. **Pesto chicken:** A ½ tsp. pesto mixed with a tbsp. low-fat mayo, shredded chicken pieces, red pepper, cherry tomatoes and green leaves.

19. **Mackerel:** Toasted wholemeal/wholegrain bread, topped with tinned mackerel in tomato sauce and green leaves.

20. **Banana:** Toast wholemeal/wholegrain bread and top with 1 tbsp. jam or 1 tsp. peanut butter. Top with mashed banana.

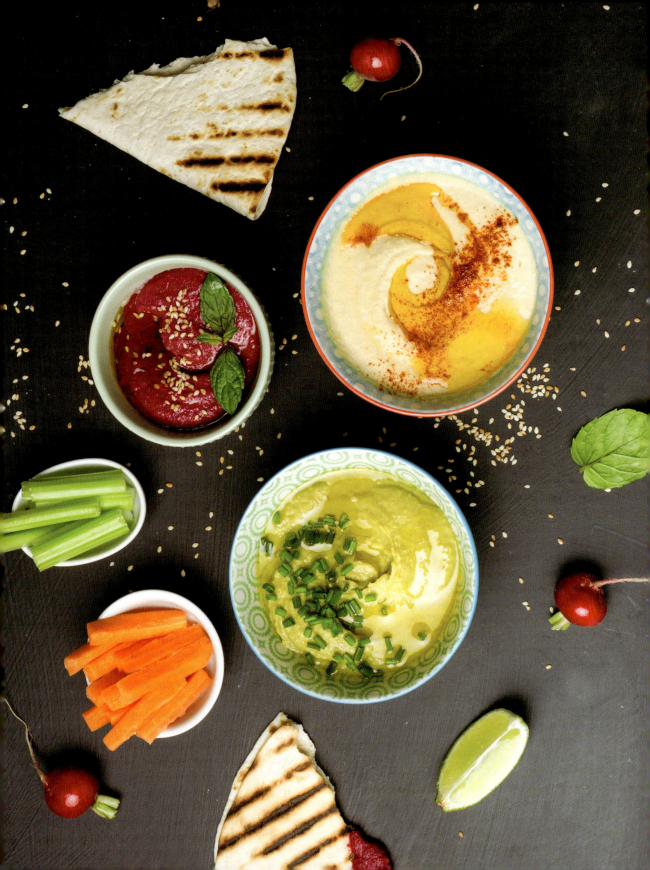

Healthy snacks

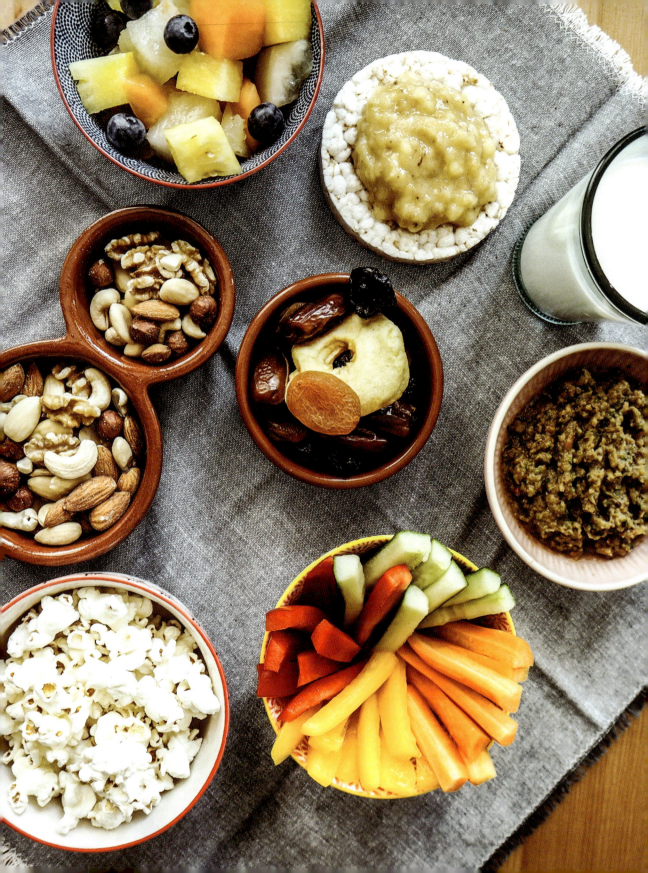

Healthy snacks

Choosing snacks that are healthy and low in calories is challenging, particularly for those on the go a lot and those who spend a lot of time outside the home. It is hugely tempting to select the high-calorie, high-fat, high-sugar options on sale at every shop checkout. These snacks often are empty calories, contributing to weight gain and providing little to no nutrients for health. Being prepared in advance and bringing healthier options with you can help minimise the temptation to snack on high-fat and high-sugar foods. Below is a list of options that are lower in calories and also snacks that provide many other important nutrients for health.

Healthy snack list

- Piece of fruit
- Handful of berries
- Fruit salad
- Fruit skewer/fruit skewer with low-fat cheese
- Chopped raw veg with hummus/healthy dip (see section 'Savoury Dips', page 151)
- ½ an avocado
- Low-fat yogurt
- Stewed fruit with yogurt
- Cup of homemade soup
- Glass of low-fat milk
- Frozen low-fat yogurt
- Bowl of homemade popcorn (not salted)
- Roasted chickpeas with spices
- Small handful of unsalted nuts, e.g. peanuts, almonds, hazelnuts, cashews, walnuts
- Small handful of dried fruit
- Overnight oats
- Small bowl of wholegrain cereal
- Small brown scone with tsp. no-added-sugar jam/nut butter
- 1 mini brown bagel with low-fat/homemade hummus/salsa/healthy dip/matchbox-size low-fat cheese/low-fat cheese spread/no-added-sugar jam
- Rice cakes/wholemeal crispbread topped with tsp. nut butter/jam
- Rice cakes/wholemeal crispbread topped with mashed banana
- Rice cakes/wholemeal crispbread topped with low-fat/homemade hummus/salsa/healthy dip
- Rice cakes/wholemeal crispbread with matchbox-size low-fat cheese/low-fat cheese spread

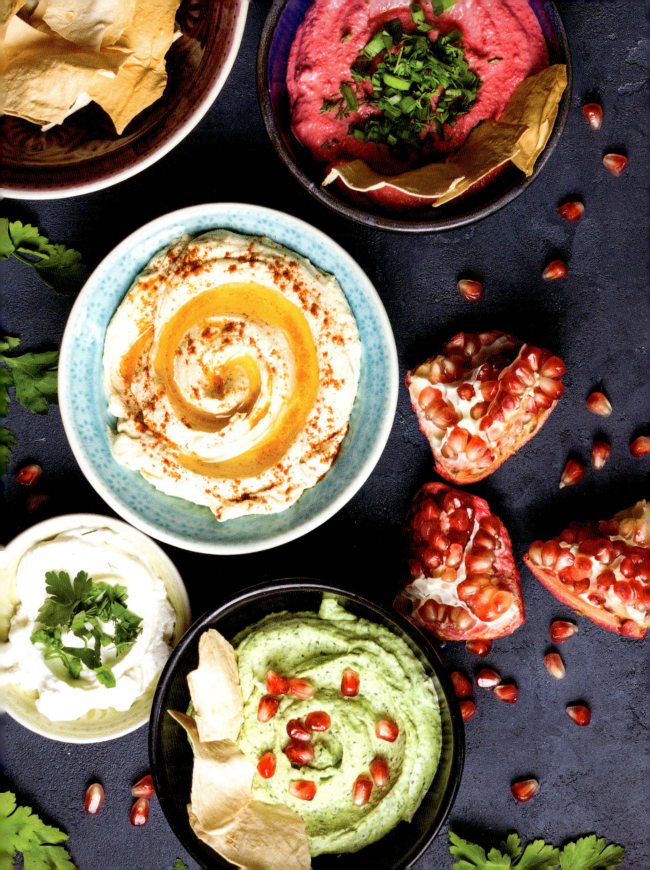

Savoury dips

Homemade tortilla chips

Vegetable crudités

Butter bean and almond dip

Easy guacamole

Red pepper hummus

Homemade tzatziki dip

Oil-free hummus

Aubergine and coriander dip

Healthy coleslaw

Spicy mango salsa

Tomato and chilli salsa

White bean dip

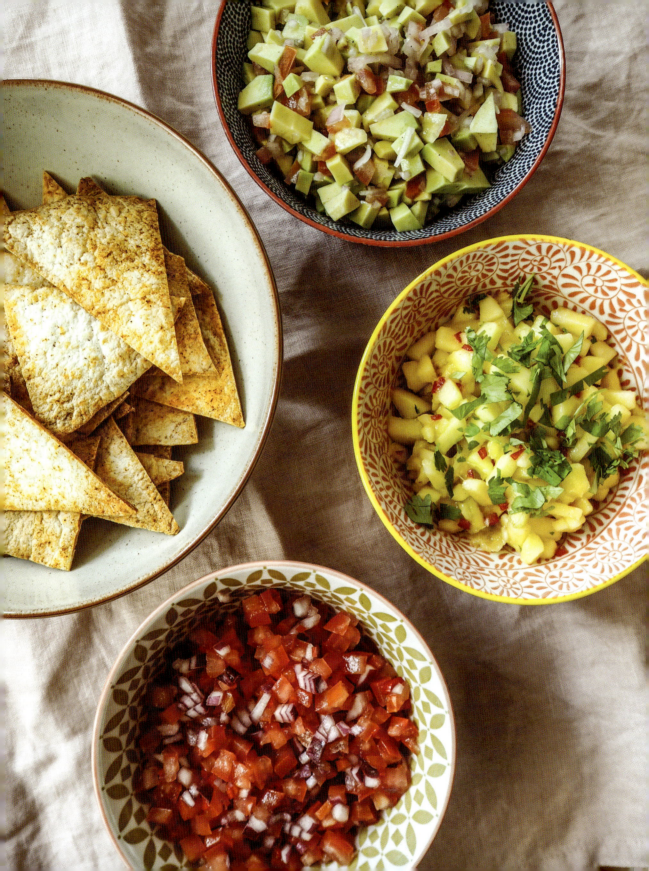

Homemade tortilla chips

🍽 **Serves:** 4 ⏱ **Prep time:** <5 mins 🍲 **Cooking time:** 10 mins

Ingredients

- 2 wholemeal tortilla wraps
- 2 tsp. olive oil or rapeseed oil
- ½ tsp. paprika
- ½ tsp. cumin

Method

1. Preheat the oven to 180°C/350°F (fan 160°C/320°F) or gas mark 4.

2. Cut the tortilla wraps into triangles and toss in the olive oil, paprika and cumin.

3. Bake in the oven until crisp.

NUTRITION INFORMATION
Amount per serving

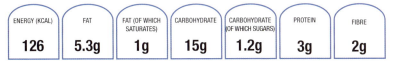

ENERGY (KCAL)	FAT	FAT (OF WHICH SATURATES)	CARBOHYDRATE	CARBOHYDRATE (OF WHICH SUGARS)	PROTEIN	FIBRE
126	5.3g	1g	15g	1.2g	3g	2g

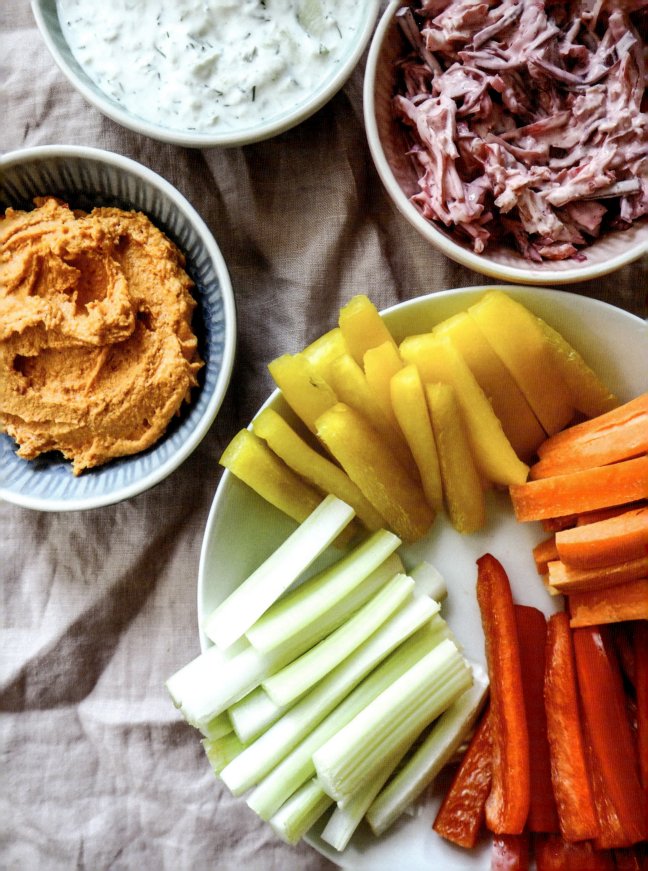

Vegetable crudités

⏱ **Prep time:** 5 mins 🍴 **Cooking time:** <5 mins

Ingredients

Selection of fresh vegetables
- Carrots, peeled and chopped into batons
- Cucumber, chopped into batons
- Celery sticks
- Selection of peppers, sliced
- Cherry tomatoes, halved
- Sugar snap peas
- Mangetout
- Broccoli

Method

1. Wash and prepare the vegetables.

2. For the peas, mangetout and broccoli, blanch by covering with boiling water for 1–2 minutes. Drain and cover with ice-cold water to prevent the vegetables from continuing to cook.

3. Arrange the vegetables on a platter and serve with a selection of dips (see pages 157–175).

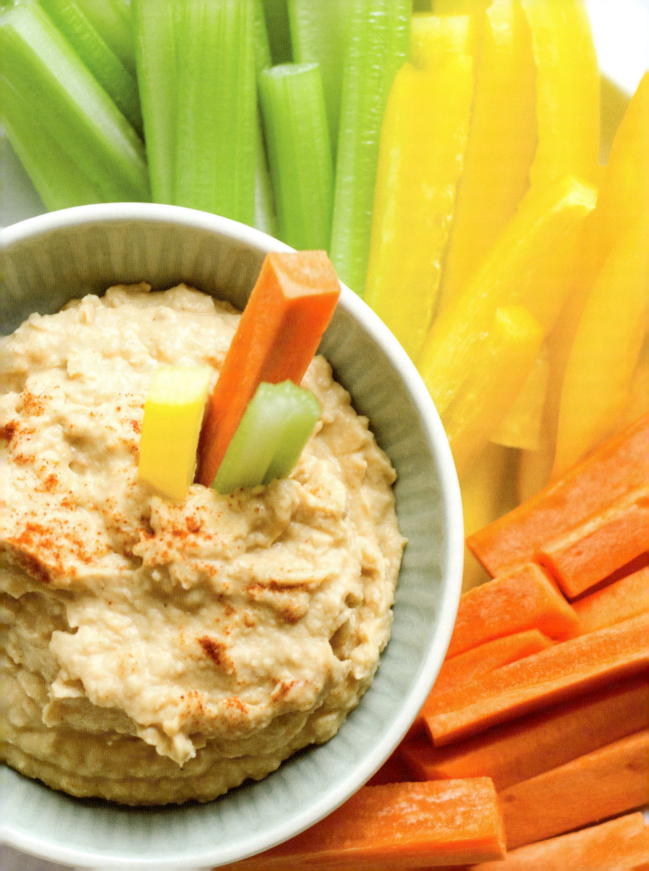

Butter bean and almond dip

🍽 **Serves:** Makes 1 bowl ⏱ **Prep time:** <5 mins

Ingredients

- 1 x 400g/14oz tin of butter beans, rinsed and drained
- 2 tbsp. almond butter
- 2 garlic cloves
- 1½ tsp. smoked paprika (to taste)
- 2½ tbsp. olive oil

Method

1. Place the butter beans, almond butter, garlic, 1 tsp. of smoked paprika and 2 tbsp. of oil into a food processor and blend until smooth.

2. Top with the remaining smoked paprika and olive oil to serve.

3. Place the dip in a bowl and serve with vegetable crudités.

NUTRITION INFORMATION
Amount per serving

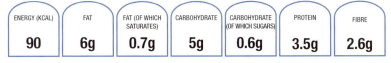

ENERGY (KCAL)	FAT	FAT (OF WHICH SATURATES)	CARBOHYDRATE	CARBOHYDRATE (OF WHICH SUGARS)	PROTEIN	FIBRE
90	6g	0.7g	5g	0.6g	3.5g	2.6g

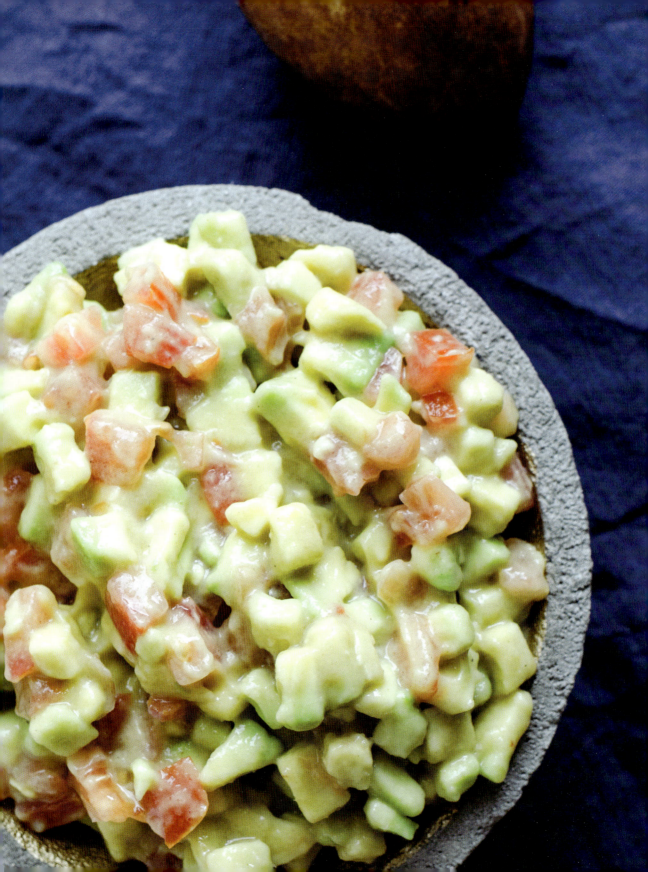

Easy guacamole

🍽 **Serves:** Makes 1 bowl ⏱ **Prep time:** 5–10 mins

Ingredients

- ½ red onion, peeled and very finely chopped
- ½ tomato, finely chopped
- 1 avocado – peeled, stone removed and cut into pieces
- 1 tsp. lime juice
- Pinch of red chilli flakes and fresh black pepper

Method

1. In a bowl, add the chopped tomato and onion. Add the lemon juice and avocado and mix well.

2. Season with pepper and chilli flakes.

NUTRITION INFORMATION
Amount per serving

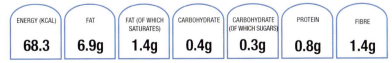

ENERGY (KCAL)	FAT	FAT (OF WHICH SATURATES)	CARBOHYDRATE	CARBOHYDRATE (OF WHICH SUGARS)	PROTEIN	FIBRE
68.3	6.9g	1.4g	0.4g	0.3g	0.8g	1.4g

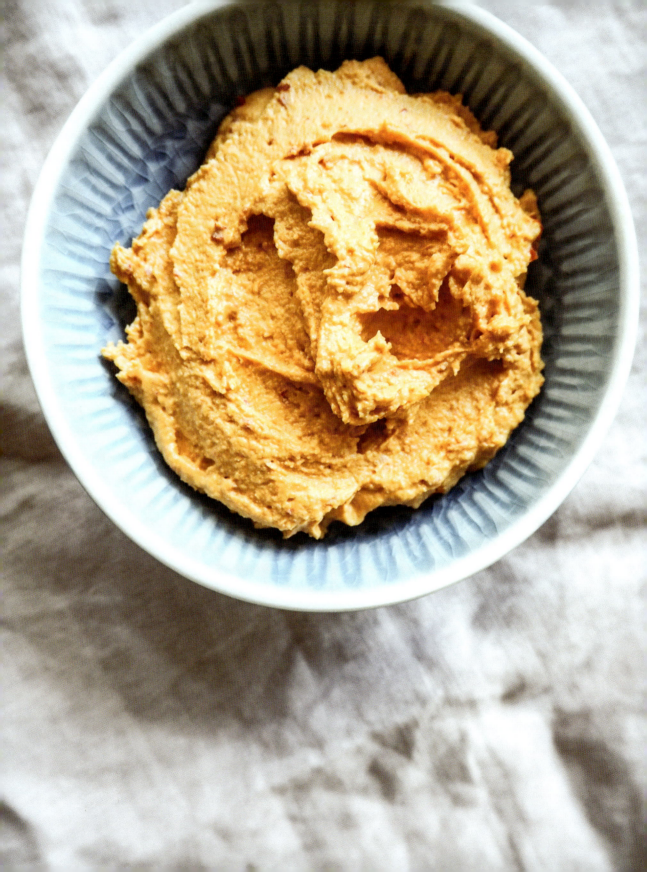

Red pepper hummus

Serves: Makes 1 bowl **Prep time:** 15 mins **Cooking time:** 15 mins (plus time to cool)

Ingredients

- 2 large red peppers (deseeded and halved lengthways)
- 1 red chilli (deseeded and halved lengthways)
- 1 tbsp. olive oil
- 2 x 400g/14oz chickpeas (drained and rinsed)
- 1 clove garlic, peeled
- 2 tbsp. tahini
- ½ lemon, juice and zest
- ½ tsp. ground cumin
- ½ tsp. ground coriander

Method

1. Preheat the grill to its hottest setting and line a baking tray with foil. Place the pepper and chilli, cut side down, on the lined tray.

2. Grill the peppers for 10 minutes or until the skins are black all over. With a pair of tongs, transfer the hot peppers to a bowl and cover tightly with cling film. The steam will help finish cooking the peppers and loosen their skins.

3. Leave to cool for 10 minutes. When the peppers are cool enough to handle, peel their skins off.

4. Place the peppers in a food processor with the other ingredients. Blend together until smooth.

5. Serve with vegetable sticks (see page 155) or a toasted wholemeal pitta bread.

6. This will store in the fridge in an airtight container for up to 3 days.

NUTRITION INFORMATION
Amount per serving

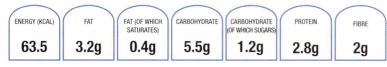

ENERGY (KCAL)	FAT	FAT (OF WHICH SATURATES)	CARBOHYDRATE	CARBOHYDRATE (OF WHICH SUGARS)	PROTEIN	FIBRE
63.5	3.2g	0.4g	5.5g	1.2g	2.8g	2g

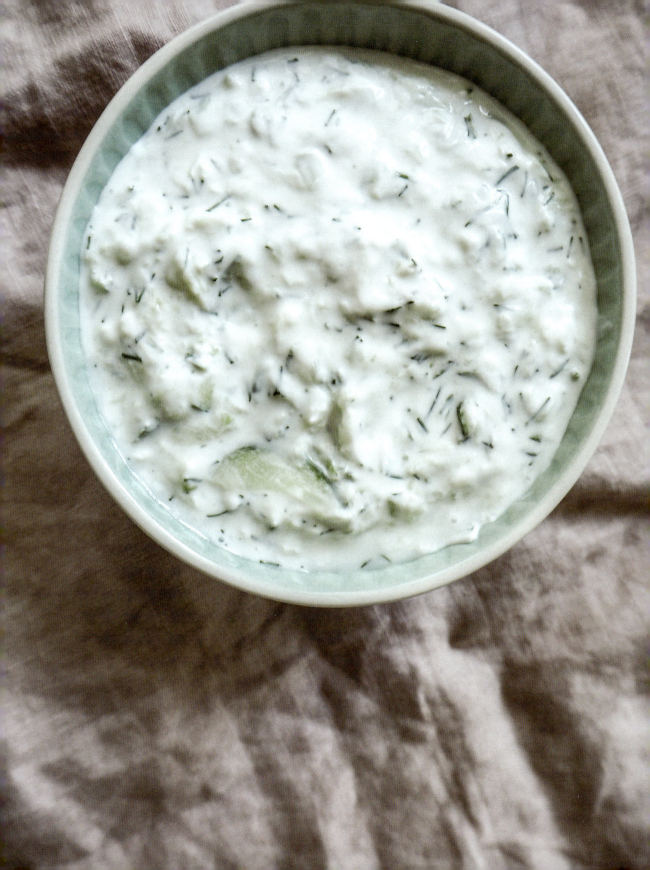

Homemade tzatziki dip

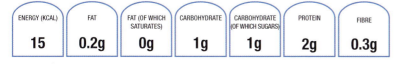 **Serves:** Makes 1 bowl ⏱ **Prep time:** <5 mins

Ingredients

- 2 cucumbers, grated
- 250g/1 cup low-fat Greek yogurt
- ½ lemon, zest and juice
- 2 cloves garlic, peeled and finely chopped
- 1 tbsp. chopped chives
- Coarse black pepper

Method

1. Put the grated cucumber into a sieve or colander and squeeze to remove excess liquid.

2. In a bowl add in the cucumber and the rest of the ingredients. Chill before serving.

NUTRITION INFORMATION
Amount per serving

ENERGY (KCAL)	FAT	FAT (OF WHICH SATURATES)	CARBOHYDRATE	CARBOHYDRATE (OF WHICH SUGARS)	PROTEIN	FIBRE
15	0.2g	0g	1g	1g	2g	0.3g

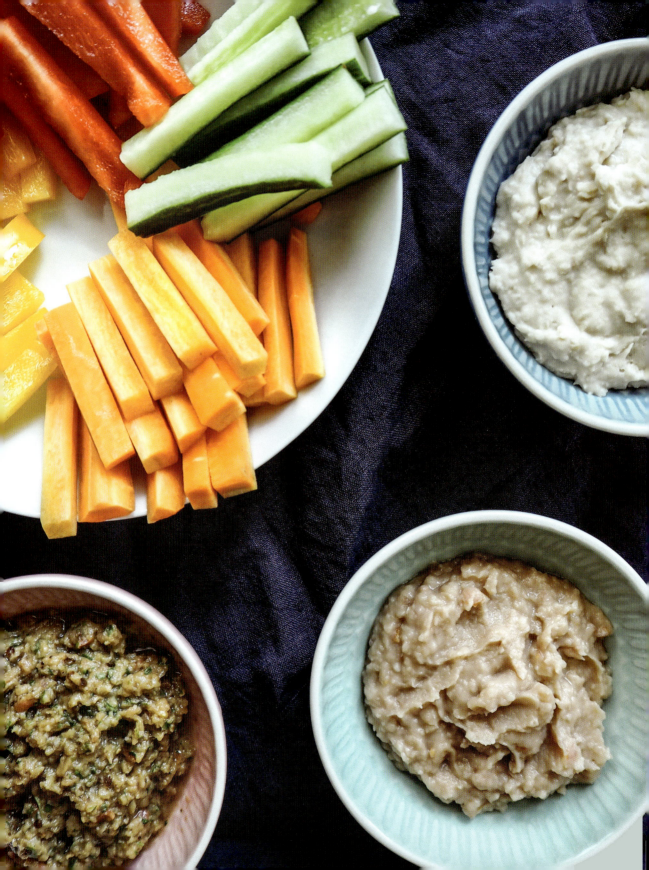

Oil-free hummus

🍽 **Serves:** Makes 1 bowl ⏱ **Prep time:** <5 mins

Ingredients

- 1 tin chickpeas
- 1 garlic clove
- 2 tbsp. almond milk
- Juice of ½ a lemon
- 2 tbsp. tahini (sesame seed paste) or ¼ cup sesame seeds
- Freshly ground black pepper

Method

1. Drain the chickpeas, rinse and set them aside.

2. Add the garlic clove to the bowl of a food processor and pulse until finely minced. Add the chickpeas and pulse until the chickpeas are finely chopped.

3. Add the almond milk, lemon juice, tahini and a twist of freshly ground black pepper. Process until the hummus is creamy and completely smooth*.

*Mixture can be thinned with a little cold water if necessary to make a smooth puree.

NUTRITION INFORMATION
Amount per serving

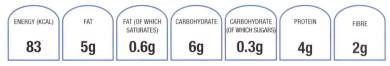

ENERGY (KCAL)	FAT	FAT (OF WHICH SATURATES)	CARBOHYDRATE	CARBOHYDRATE (OF WHICH SUGARS)	PROTEIN	FIBRE
83	5g	0.6g	6g	0.3g	4g	2g

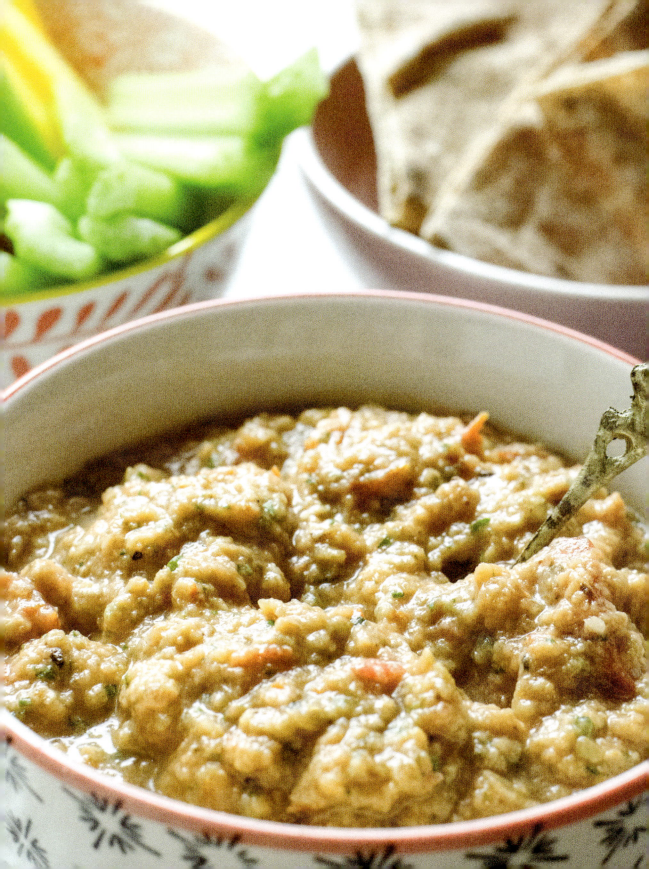

Aubergine and coriander dip

🍽 **Serves:** Makes 1 large bowl ⏱ **Prep time:** 10 mins 🍵 **Cooking time:** 45 mins

Ingredients

- 2 medium aubergines
- 500g/18oz/5 large tomatoes
- 3 spring onions, roughly chopped
- 50g/2oz/1 large bag fresh coriander
- 2 cloves garlic
- Juice of ½ a lemon
- Pepper to season
- Raw carrot, pepper, celery and crunchy pitta pieces for serving

Method

1. Preheat the oven to 180°C/350°F (fan 160°C/320°F) or gas mark 4.

2. Prick the aubergines all over with a fork. Place them on a baking tray and bake in the oven for 45 minutes to1 hour until they collapse and are soft inside. Allow them to cool and then peel and chop the flesh.

3. Meanwhile prepare the other ingredients. Chop the tomatoes and spring onions. Remove the coriander leaves from the stalks and chop. Peel and chop the garlic.

4. Combine all the ingredients in a blender/food processor and blend to a rough sauce. Transfer to a serving bowl and serve with raw vegetables or wholemeal pitta bread pieces.

NUTRITION INFORMATION
Amount per serving

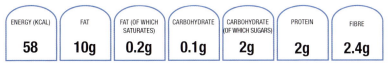

ENERGY (KCAL)	FAT	FAT (OF WHICH SATURATES)	CARBOHYDRATE	CARBOHYDRATE (OF WHICH SUGARS)	PROTEIN	FIBRE
58	10g	0.2g	0.1g	2g	2g	2.4g

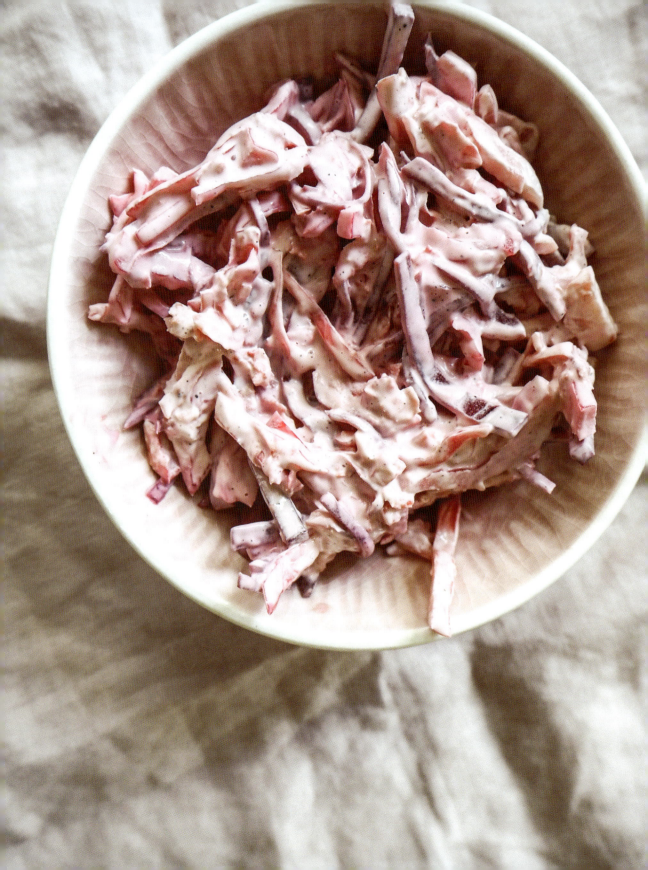

Healthy coleslaw

🍽 **Serves:** Makes 1 large bowl ⏱ **Prep time:** 10 mins

Ingredients

- 2 carrots, peeled and grated
- 1 small raw beetroot, peeled and grated
- ¼ head white or red cabbage, finely sliced
- 1 medium apple, skin on and grated
- 2–3 tbsp. freshly chopped parsley or chives

Dressing:
- 1 tsp. brown sugar
- Juice of ½ a lime
- 3 tbsp. low-fat natural yogurt
- Pinch of salt and black pepper
- Toasted seeds to serve – e.g. pumpkin, sunflower

Method

1. Combine the prepared vegetables in a large bowl.

2. Dissolve the sugar in the lime juice. Mix with the natural yogurt. Add a pinch of salt and black pepper.

3. Toast the seeds by heating them on a dry frying pan over a medium heat until lightly golden.

4. Pour the dressing over the vegetables and mix well. Garnish with toasted seeds and freshly chopped parsley or chives.

NUTRITION INFORMATION
Amount per serving

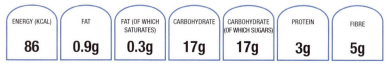

ENERGY (KCAL)	FAT	FAT (OF WHICH SATURATES)	CARBOHYDRATE	CARBOHYDRATE (OF WHICH SUGARS)	PROTEIN	FIBRE
86	0.9g	0.3g	17g	17g	3g	5g

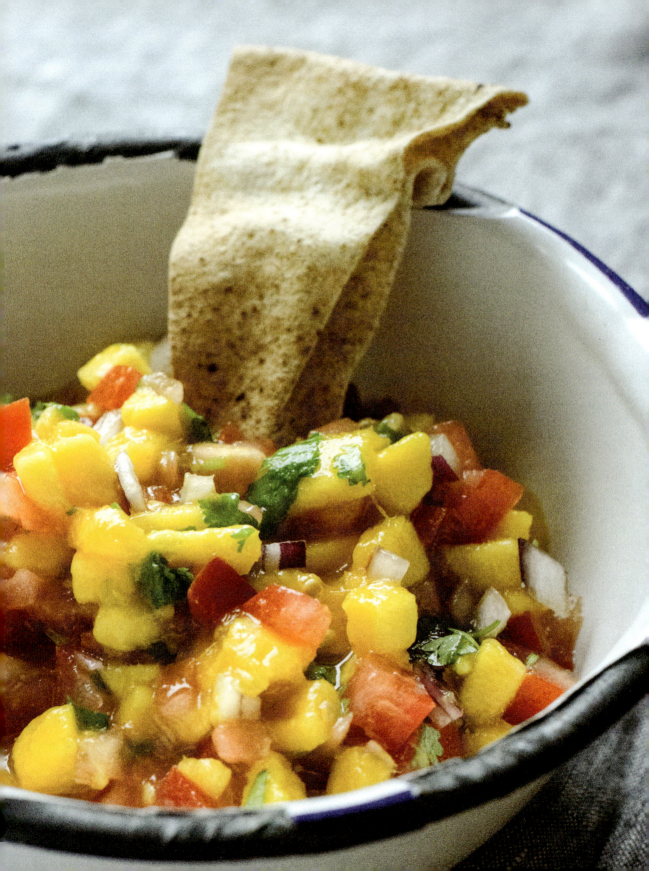

Spicy mango salsa

Serves: Makes 1 bowl **Prep time:** 5–10 mins

Ingredients

- 1 ripe mango, peeled and diced
- 4 ripe tomatoes, skinned and chopped
- 1 small red chilli, seeds removed and chopped
- Juice of 1 lime
- Ground black pepper
- 3 tbsp. freshly chopped coriander leaves

Method

1. Mix the chopped ingredients together. Season to taste and store in the refrigerator until required.

NUTRITION INFORMATION
Amount per serving

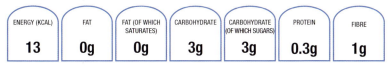

ENERGY (KCAL)	FAT	FAT (OF WHICH SATURATES)	CARBOHYDRATE	CARBOHYDRATE (OF WHICH SUGARS)	PROTEIN	FIBRE
13	0g	0g	3g	3g	0.3g	1g

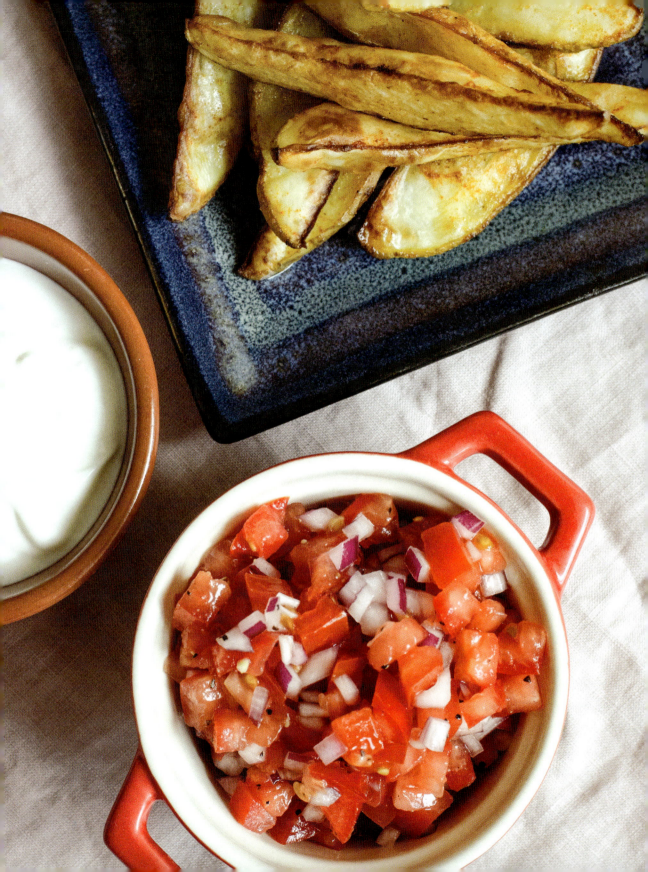

Tomato and chilli salsa

🍽 **Serves:** Makes 1 bowl ⏱ **Prep time:** 5–10 mins

Ingredients

- 2 large tomatoes, finely chopped
- ½ a red onion, peeled and finely chopped
- 1 small chilli, finely chopped
- Juice of ½ a lime
- Pepper
- Pinch of sugar

Method

1. Mix all the ingredients together.
2. Taste and correct the seasoning.

NUTRITION INFORMATION
Amount per serving

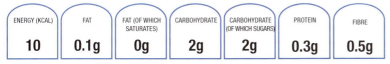

ENERGY (KCAL)	FAT	FAT (OF WHICH SATURATES)	CARBOHYDRATE	CARBOHYDRATE (OF WHICH SUGARS)	PROTEIN	FIBRE
10	0.1g	0g	2g	2g	0.3g	0.5g

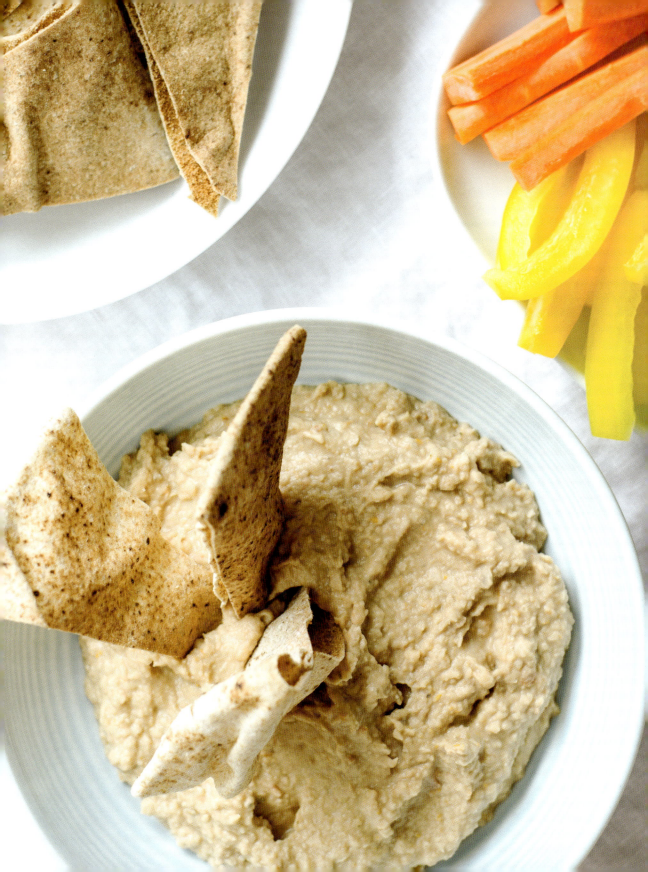

White bean dip

🍽 **Serves:** Makes 1 bowl ⏱ **Prep time:** 5–10 mins

Ingredients

- 1 tin cannellini beans, drained
- 4 sun-dried tomatoes
- ½ clove garlic
- ½ tbsp. balsamic vinegar
- 2 tbsp. olive oil
- Pinch black pepper
- Cold water to make a smooth puree

Method

1. Blitz all the ingredients with a hand blender or food processor. Add extra water and blitz again if the consistency is too thick. Empty into a bowl and serve with toasted pitta and vegetable sticks like carrot, pepper and celery (see page 155).

NUTRITION INFORMATION
Amount per serving

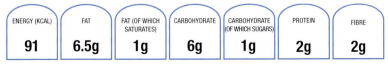

ENERGY (KCAL)	FAT	FAT (OF WHICH SATURATES)	CARBOHYDRATE	CARBOHYDRATE (OF WHICH SUGARS)	PROTEIN	FIBRE
91	6.5g	1g	6g	1g	2g	2g

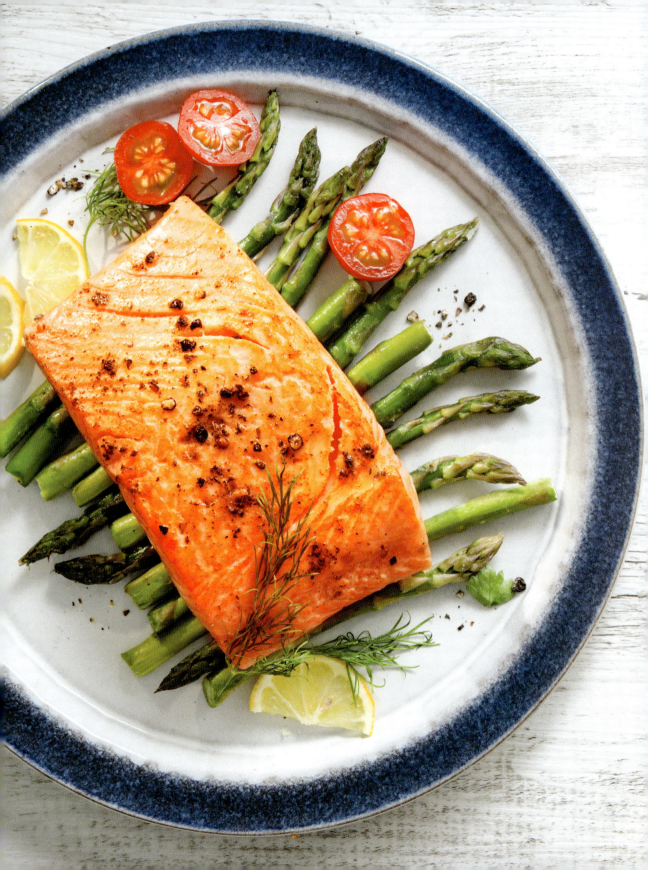

Main meals

Red meat

Beef burgers

Beef stew

Beef stroganoff

Chilli con carne

Italian meatballs with pasta

Lamb tagine

Healthy lasagne

Shepherd's pie

Spaghetti bolognese

Spiced pork tray bake

Steak with salsa verde

Sweet and sour pork

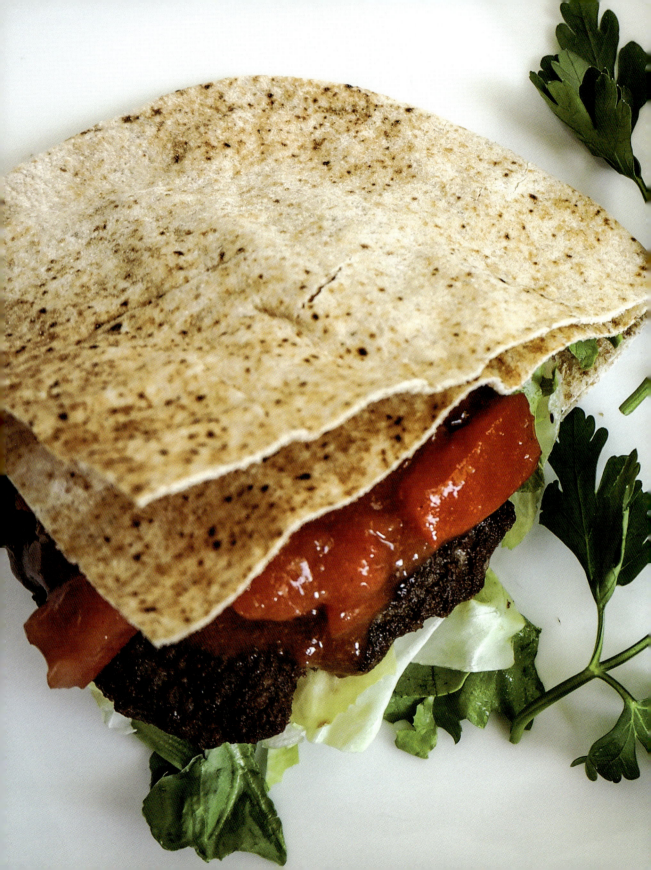

Beef burgers

🍽 **Serves:** 4 ⏱ **Prep time:** 10 mins 🍲 **Cooking time:** 15 mins

Ingredients

- 2 slices of wholegrain bread
- 100ml/½ cup low-fat milk
- 350g/12oz lean minced beef
- 1 tbsp. chopped parsley
- 1 egg, beaten
- Pinch of pepper
- 3 tbsp. olive oil
- 8 vine tomatoes
- 1 tsp. Tabasco sauce
- 4 small round wholemeal pittas/ wholemeal burger buns
- Mixed salad leaves to add to pitta plus large side salad to serve

Method

1. Remove the crusts from the bread and blitz to make breadcrumbs. Add the milk and mix well.

2. Add the minced beef, chopped parsley, egg and pepper to the bowl and mix.

3. Shape the mixture into four burgers. Heat the oil in a pan and cook the burgers until golden brown on each side and cooked through, about 10 minutes.

4. Chop the tomatoes into small pieces and add Tabasco sauce to taste.

5. Place the beef burgers and mixed leaves in a toasted burger bun/pitta pocket. Serve with tomato pieces and a large salad on the side.

NUTRITION INFORMATION
Amount per serving

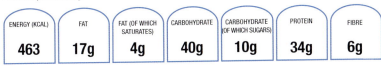

ENERGY (KCAL)	FAT	FAT (OF WHICH SATURATES)	CARBOHYDRATE	CARBOHYDRATE (OF WHICH SUGARS)	PROTEIN	FIBRE
463	17g	4g	40g	10g	34g	6g

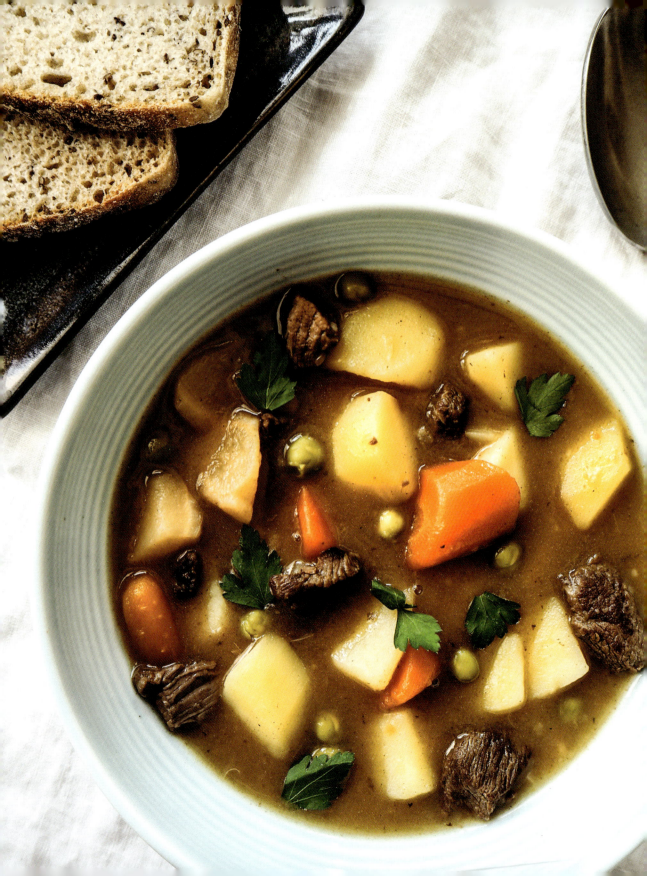

Beef stew

🍽 **Serves:** 4 ⏱ **Prep time:** 20 mins 🍲 **Cooking time:** 1½–2 hours

Ingredients

- 2 tbsp. vegetable oil
- 450g/1lb stewing beef, fat trimmed off
- 5 carrots, peeled and roughly chopped
- 2 small onions, peeled and roughly chopped
- 1 parsnip, peeled and roughly chopped
- 1.2 litre/5 cups homemade beef stock or 2 beef stock cubes dissolved in 1 litre/4¼ cups of warm water
- 40g/⅓ cup flour
- 3 dessertspoons of frozen peas
- 4 potatoes, peeled and chopped

Method

1. Fry the beef pieces in 1 tbsp. of oil until browned.

2. Remove the meat from the frying pan and place in an extra-large saucepan.

3. Next, lightly fry the chopped onions, carrots and parsnips in 1 tbsp. of oil in the same frying pan.

4. Remove the vegetables from the frying pan and place in the saucepan with the meat.

5. Add a few spoons of stock to the frying pan, then sprinkle in the flour and stir well to combine.

6. Add the remaining stock and continue stirring over a low heat.

7. Add the thickened stock to the saucepan with the meat and vegetables. Cook gently over a low heat for 1–1½ hours until the meat is tender.

8. Add the washed and peeled potatoes to the stew 30 minutes before the end of the cooking time.

9. Add the frozen peas to the stew 10 minutes before the end of cooking time. This may also be cooked as a casserole in the oven.

NUTRITION INFORMATION
Amount per serving

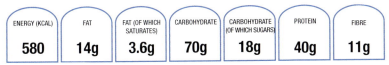

ENERGY (KCAL)	FAT	FAT (OF WHICH SATURATES)	CARBOHYDRATE	CARBOHYDRATE (OF WHICH SUGARS)	PROTEIN	FIBRE
580	14g	3.6g	70g	18g	40g	11g

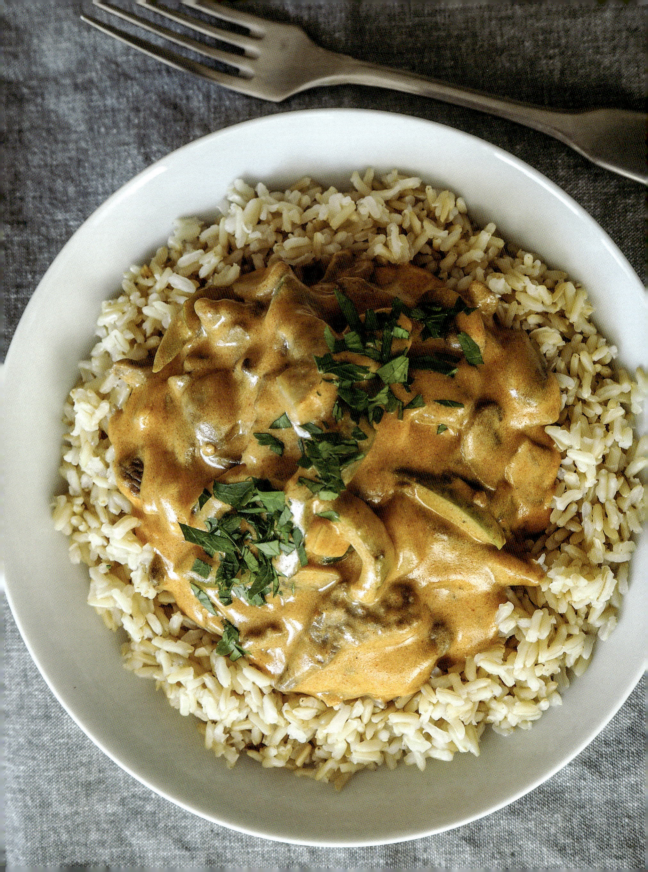

Beef stroganoff

🍽 **Serves:** 4 ⏱ **Prep time:** 10 mins 🍲 **Cooking time:** 15–20 mins

Ingredients

- 240g/1 cup wholegrain/brown rice (~150g/¾ cup cooked per person)
- 1 tbsp. vegetable oil
- 1 small onion, peeled and sliced
- 3 cloves of garlic, crushed
- 1 heaped tsp. paprika
- 1 green pepper, sliced
- 300g/4 cups mushrooms
- 400g/14oz sirloin steak, fat removed and cut into thin strips
- 2 tbsp. red wine vinegar
- 150ml/½ cup beef stock
- 3–4 heaped tbsp. low-fat/fat-free crème fraiche

Method

1. Cook the rice as per packet instructions.

2. Heat the oil in a pan and fry the onion until soft. Add the garlic and paprika and cook for 1–2 minutes until fragrant. Add the pepper and mushrooms and fry for 5–8 minutes until softened.

3. Add the beef and cook for 2–3 minutes, depending on how rare you like it.

4. Add the vinegar, boil to reduce until almost evaporated, then pour over the stock and bubble for a few minutes until thickened slightly. Remove from the heat and stir in the crème fraiche.

5. Serve on a bed of cooked brown rice.

NUTRITION INFORMATION
Amount per serving

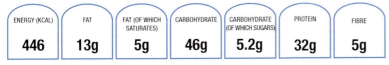

ENERGY (KCAL)	FAT	FAT (OF WHICH SATURATES)	CARBOHYDRATE	CARBOHYDRATE (OF WHICH SUGARS)	PROTEIN	FIBRE
446	13g	5g	46g	5.2g	32g	5g

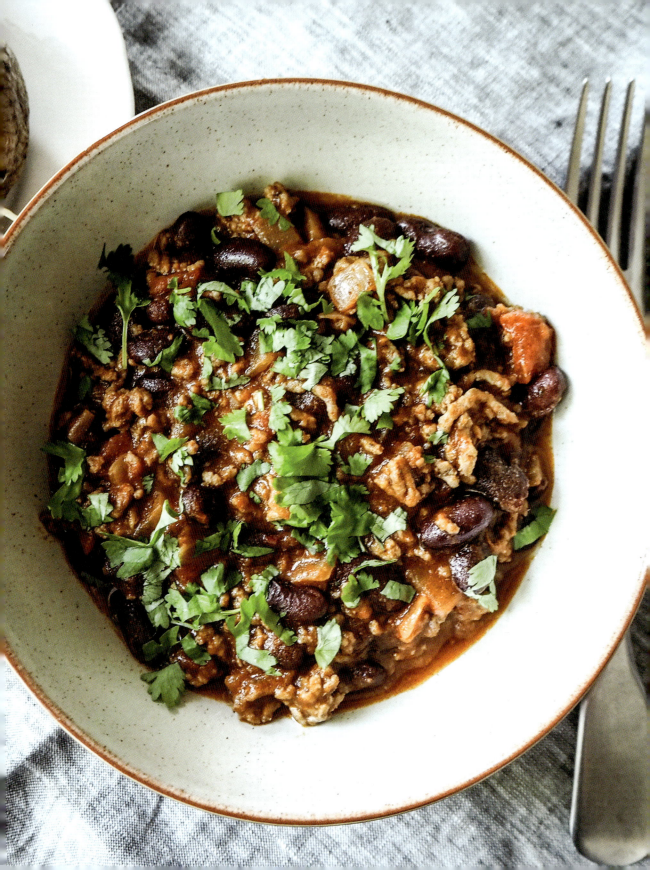

Chilli con carne

🍽 **Serves:** 4 ⏱ **Prep time:** 10 mins 🍲 **Cooking time:** 35–40 mins

Ingredients

- 1 tsp. olive oil or rapeseed oil
- 1 onion, finely chopped
- 500g/18oz lean beef mince (<5% fat/95% fat-free)
- 2 garlic cloves, finely chopped/crushed
- 2 fresh chillies, deseeded and chopped
- 2 tsp. ground cumin
- 1 tsp. ground coriander
- 1 tsp. paprika
- Pinch cayenne pepper
- 400g/14oz tin chopped tomatoes
- 1 level tbsp. tomato puree
- 300ml/1¼ cups beef stock
- Freshly ground black pepper
- 400g/14oz tin red kidney beans, drained
- Chopped fresh coriander leaves to garnish

Serve with a baked potato (1 large per person) or brown rice (~60g/¼ cup raw/150g/¾ cup cooked brown rice per person).

Method

1. Fry the onions gently over a low heat in 1 tsp. oil until softened. Add the mince and stir-fry for 5–6 minutes.

2. Add the garlic, chillies and all of the spices and continue to fry for 2–3 minutes.

3. Add the tinned tomatoes, tomato puree and stock. Stir well and bring to the boil. Reduce the heat and simmer gently for 20 minutes, until the liquid is slightly reduced.

4. Add the drained kidney beans. Heat through gently for about 5 minutes.

5. Season with pepper and serve garnished with chopped coriander leaves.

6. Serve with a baked potato or a portion of cooked brown rice.

NUTRITION INFORMATION
Amount per serving

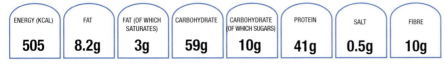

ENERGY (KCAL)	FAT	FAT (OF WHICH SATURATES)	CARBOHYDRATE	CARBOHYDRATE (OF WHICH SUGARS)	PROTEIN	SALT	FIBRE
505	8.2g	3g	59g	10g	41g	0.5g	10g

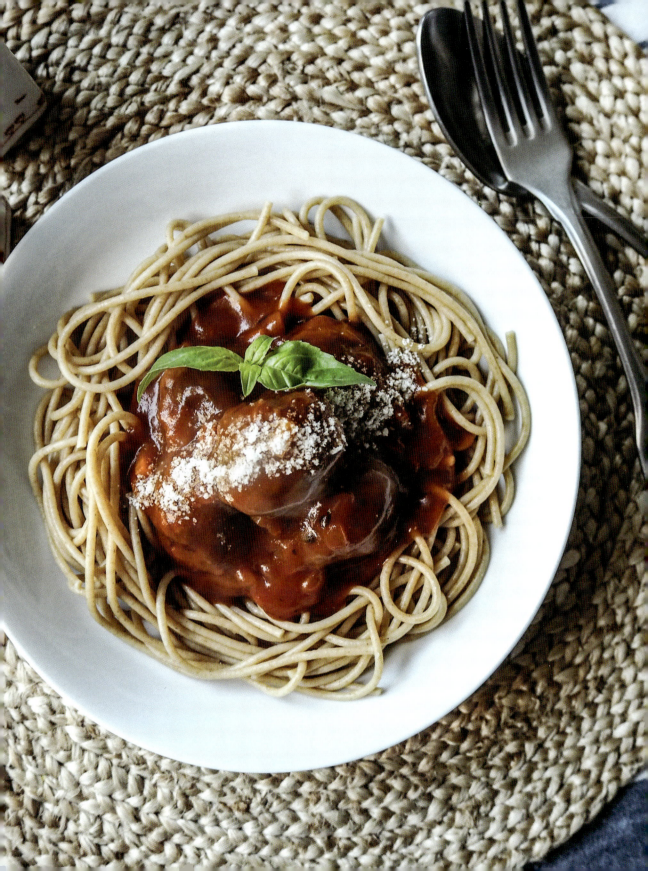

Italian meatballs with pasta

🍽 **Serves:** 6 ⏱ **Prep time:** 25 mins 🍲 **Cooking time:** 30 mins

Ingredients

Meatballs:
- 2 tbsp. olive oil
- 1 large onion, finely chopped
- 500g/18oz lean minced beef* (<5% fat/95% fat-free)
- 50g/½ cup breadcrumbs
- 1 egg, beaten
- 1–2 tsp. thyme or oregano
- Freshly ground black pepper
- Zest of ½ a lemon

Tomato sauce:
- 1 tbsp. olive oil
- 1 large onion, peeled and finely chopped
- 1 small carrot, peeled and very finely chopped or grated
- 2 sticks celery, very finely chopped
- 2 cloves garlic, peeled and crushed
- 2 tins tomatoes
- Pinch nutmeg

Serve with cooked brown pasta (~150g/¾ cup cooked (60g/½ cup raw) per person).

Method

1. Sweat the onion in a little olive oil until soft. Allow to cool.

2. Mix all ingredients (except olive oil) together and form into meatballs. Cover and allow to chill in the fridge.

3. To make the sauce, heat the oil in a pan. Cook the onions, carrot and celery gently until soft but not coloured.

4. Add the garlic, tomatoes and nutmeg. Simmer for about 30 minutes until thickened.

5. Heat the remaining olive oil in a pan and fry the meatballs until lightly browned.

6. Pour tomato sauce over the meatballs and simmer gently until cooked through.

7. Serve with a portion of cooked brown pasta.

*As a variation of this recipe, the minced beef can be substituted with minced turkey.

NUTRITION INFORMATION
Amount per serving

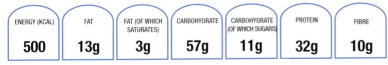

ENERGY (KCAL)	FAT	FAT (OF WHICH SATURATES)	CARBOHYDRATE	CARBOHYDRATE (OF WHICH SUGARS)	PROTEIN	FIBRE
500	13g	3g	57g	11g	32g	10g

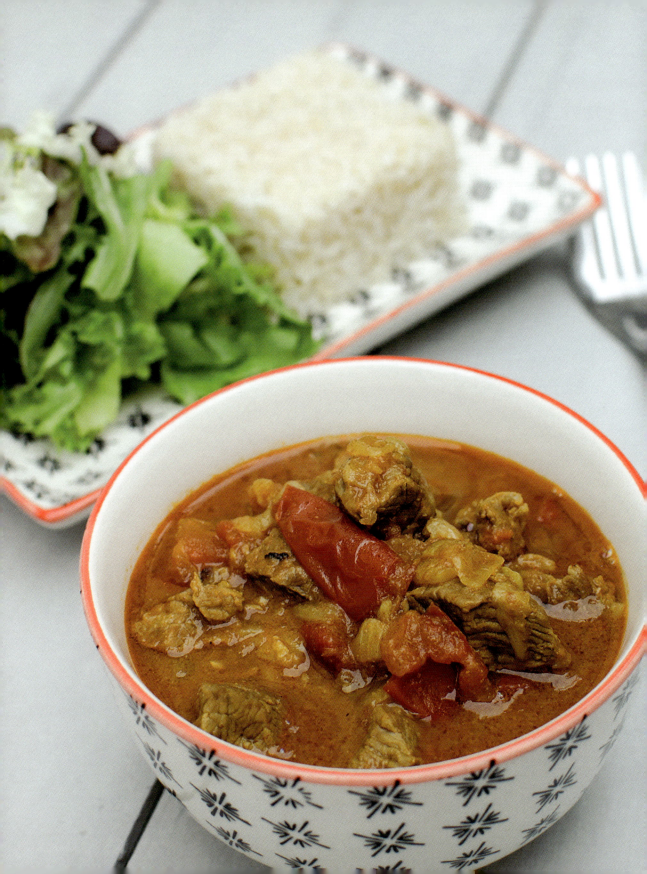

Lamb tagine

🍽 **Serves:** 4 ⏱ **Prep time:** 20 mins 🍲 **Cooking time:** 2 hours

Ingredients

- 1 tbsp. olive oil
- 2 cloves garlic, chopped
- 1 large onion, peeled and finely chopped
- 2 small carrots, grated
- 200g/7oz of butternut squash, peeled and cubed
- 1 heaped tbsp. grated ginger
- 1 tbsp. ground cumin or cumin seeds, crushed
- 1 tbsp. coriander seeds, crushed
- 1 tbsp. ground ginger
- Freshly ground black pepper
- 450g/1lb leg/shoulder of lamb (lean meat, fat trimmed), cubed
- 1 tbsp. tomato puree
- 1 x 400g/14oz tin tomatoes
- 1 tbsp. honey
- 1 x 400g/14oz tin of chickpeas, drained
- 240g/1 cup (raw weight: 4 servings) wholegrain brown rice
- Fresh coriander to garnish

Method

1. Preheat the oven to 160°C/320°F (fan 140°C/280°F) or gas mark 3.

2. Heat the oil in a large casserole dish and add the onion, carrots, butternut squash, garlic, ginger and spices. Cover and cook on a low heat for 10 minutes.

3. Add the lamb, chickpeas, tomatoes, tomato puree and honey. Mix well and transfer to the hot oven for 90 minutes. After 45 minutes, remove the lid.

4. Cook the rice as per packet instructions. Serve each portion of tagine on a bed of cooked wholegrain brown rice and garnish with coriander.

NUTRITION INFORMATION
Amount per serving

ENERGY (KCAL)	FAT	FAT (OF WHICH SATURATES)	CARBOHYDRATE	CARBOHYDRATE (OF WHICH SUGARS)	PROTEIN	FIBRE
564	14g	1g	70g	19g	35g	12g

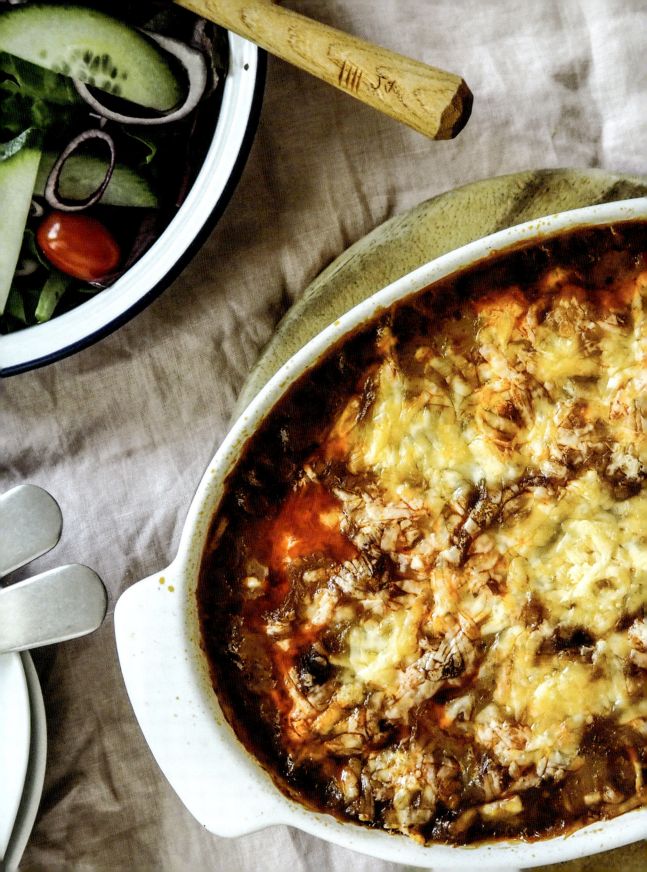

Healthy lasagne

🍽 **Serves:** 6 ⏱ **Prep time:** 20 mins 🍲 **Cooking time:** 60 mins

Ingredients

- 1 tbsp. extra virgin olive oil
- 1 large onion, peeled and finely chopped
- 3 medium carrots, peeled and finely chopped or grated
- 1 red pepper, deseeded and finely chopped
- 2 celery sticks, finely chopped
- 2 garlic cloves, peeled and crushed
- 400g/14oz lean minced beef (<5% fat)
- 150g/2 cups chopped button mushrooms, chopped
- 2 tbsp. tomato puree
- 680ml/24oz jar of passata
- 2 tsp. dried mixed herbs
- Freshly ground black pepper
- 7–10 sheets wholewheat lasagne sheets
- 50g/½ cup grated low-fat cheese

For the white sauce:
- 500ml/2 cups skimmed/low-fat milk
- 2 tbsp. cornflour
- Pinch nutmeg

Serve with large green side salad.

Method

1. Heat the oil in a large, lidded saucepan over a low heat. Add the onion and fry gently for 5 minutes. Add the carrots, red pepper, celery and garlic and cook for a further 5 minutes, or until the onion is soft and just beginning to colour.

2. Turn up the heat a little, then add the beef mince and cook, stirring until browned and crumbly. Add the mushrooms and cook for 1 more minute, then drain off any fat from the meat.

3. Stir in the passata, tomato puree and dried herbs. Bring to the boil, then gently simmer over a low heat for 20 minutes, stirring occasionally. Season with black pepper.

4. Preheat the oven to 200°C/400°F (fan 180°C/350°F) or gas mark 6.

5. To make the white sauce, mix the cornflour with a little milk to make a smooth paste. Add more milk until all the cornflour has been dissolved and it is a runny consistency. Now put the cornflour mixture along with the remaining milk into a medium-sized saucepan. Over a medium heat, bring to the boil while stirring continuously. Simmer for 2 minutes and stir in the nutmeg. Once the sauce has reached a custard consistency, take it off the heat.

6. Spoon half the meat sauce over the base of an ovenproof dish or roasting tin. Cover with a layer of lasagne, then spoon over the remaining meat sauce and cover with another layer of pasta.

7. Pour over the white sauce to cover the lasagne completely. Scatter over the grated cheese.

8. Bake for 30 minutes, or until the lasagne is bubbling and the top is lightly browned.

9. Serve with a large side salad.

NUTRITION INFORMATION
Amount per serving

ENERGY (KCAL)	FAT	FAT (OF WHICH SATURATES)	CARBOHYDRATE	CARBOHYDRATE (OF WHICH SUGARS)	PROTEIN	SALT	FIBRE
430	8g	3g	57g	23g	30g	0.9g	11g

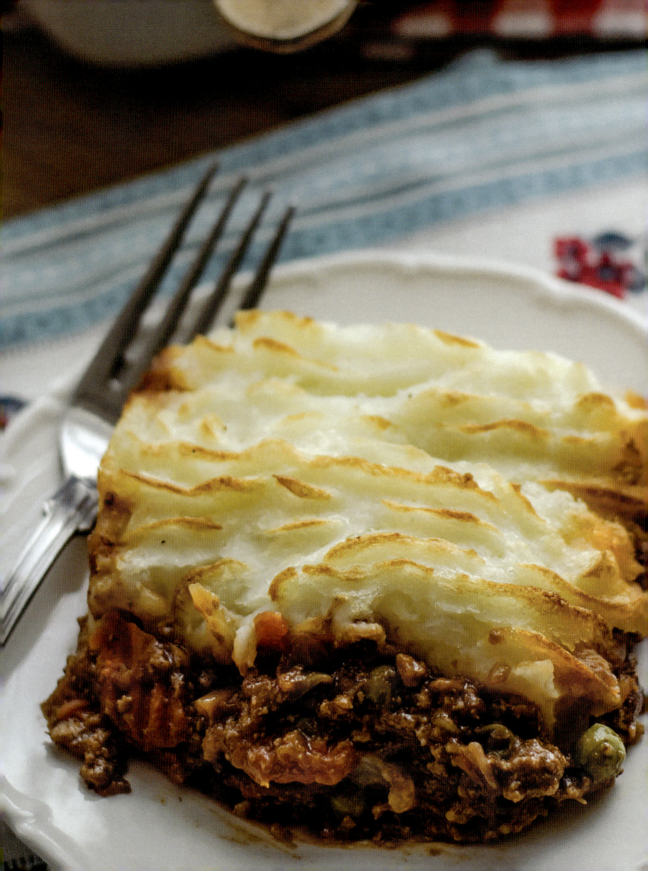

Shepherd's pie

🍽 **Serves:** 6 ⏱ **Prep time:** 20 mins 🍲 **Cooking time:** 1 hour

Ingredients

- 3 carrots, peeled and diced
- 800g/1¾lb potatoes, peeled and quartered
- 250g/9oz broccoli florets
- 50ml/¼ cup semi-skimmed/low-fat milk
- 1 tbsp. olive oil
- 1 small onion, peeled and diced
- 2 cloves of garlic, peeled and crushed
- 400g/14oz lean minced beef (<5% fat)
- 300g/4 cups mushrooms, peeled and cut in half
- 1 beef or vegetable stock cube dissolved in 350ml/1½ cups of boiling water or 350ml/1½ cups homemade stock
- 1 tbsp. tomato puree
- 2 tbsp. Worcestershire sauce
- 2 tsp. cornflour mixed with 20ml/2 dessert spoons water
- 75g/½ cup frozen peas
- 50g/½ cup low-fat cheese, grated

Method

1. Preheat the oven to 180°C/350°F (fan 160°C/320°F) or gas mark 4.

2. In a steamer place the carrots and potatoes and steam until soft (approximately 15 minutes). With 5 minutes to go, add the broccoli and steam. Set the carrots and broccoli aside and drain and mash the potatoes with the milk.

3. Meanwhile, add the olive oil to a pan and cook the onion and garlic until softened. Add the mince and fry until browned (approximately 15 minutes) and drain off any excess fat from the pan.

4. Remove the meat from the pan and fry the mushrooms in the pan (2 minutes). Add the mince back into the pan and then add the stock, tomato puree and Worcestershire sauce and bring to the boil, stirring all the time. Add the peas, carrots and broccoli. Thicken the liquid by adding cornflour and water to the pan.

5. Transfer the meat and vegetables to a casserole dish.

6. Spoon the mash on top of the meat and smooth with a knife or fork to form a pattern on top.

7. Sprinkle the top with low-fat cheese.

8. Bake in the preheated oven for 25 minutes until golden on top.

NUTRITION INFORMATION
Amount per serving

ENERGY (KCAL)	FAT	FAT (OF WHICH SATURATES)	CARBOHYDRATE	CARBOHYDRATE (OF WHICH SUGARS)	PROTEIN	FIBRE
440	10g	4g	49g	13g	36g	10g

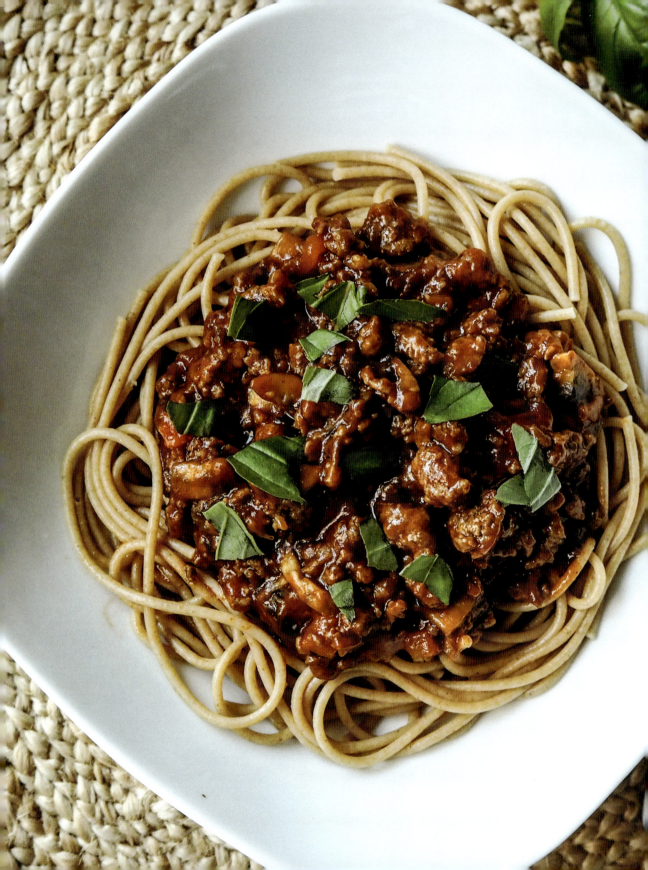

Spaghetti bolognese

Serves: 4 **Prep time:** 15 mins **Cooking time:** 30 mins

Ingredients

- 1 tbsp. sunflower oil
- 1 large onion, peeled and finely chopped
- 2 cloves garlic, peeled and chopped
- 400g/14oz lean minced beef (<5% fat)
- 200g/2½ cups mushrooms, sliced
- 2 carrots, grated
- 600ml/2½ cups passata or 400g/14oz tinned tomatoes and 200ml/¾ cup low-salt vegetable stock
- 2 tbsp. tomato puree
- 1 tbsp. dried oregano*
- Season with black pepper
- 240g/8½oz wholewheat spaghetti, raw
- Basil leaves to garnish

*Alternative to oregano is 1 tbsp smoked paprika.

Method

1. Heat the oil in a large frying pan over a medium heat.

2. Add the onion, garlic and mince and fry, stirring occasionally, until the mince is browned and the onions softened.

3. Add the mushrooms and grated carrots, cook for one minute, then add the passata/tinned tomatoes and vegetable stock, tomato puree, oregano and freshly ground black pepper. Stir well and bring to the boil, then reduce the heat to simmer for 15–20 minutes, until the sauce has thickened.

4. Cook the wholewheat spaghetti according to the packet instructions, then drain.

5. Mix the sauce through the cooked spaghetti and serve garnished with fresh basil leaves.

NUTRITION INFORMATION
Amount per serving

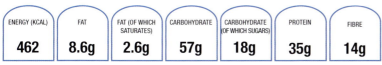

ENERGY (KCAL)	FAT	FAT (OF WHICH SATURATES)	CARBOHYDRATE	CARBOHYDRATE (OF WHICH SUGARS)	PROTEIN	FIBRE
462	8.6g	2.6g	57g	18g	35g	14g

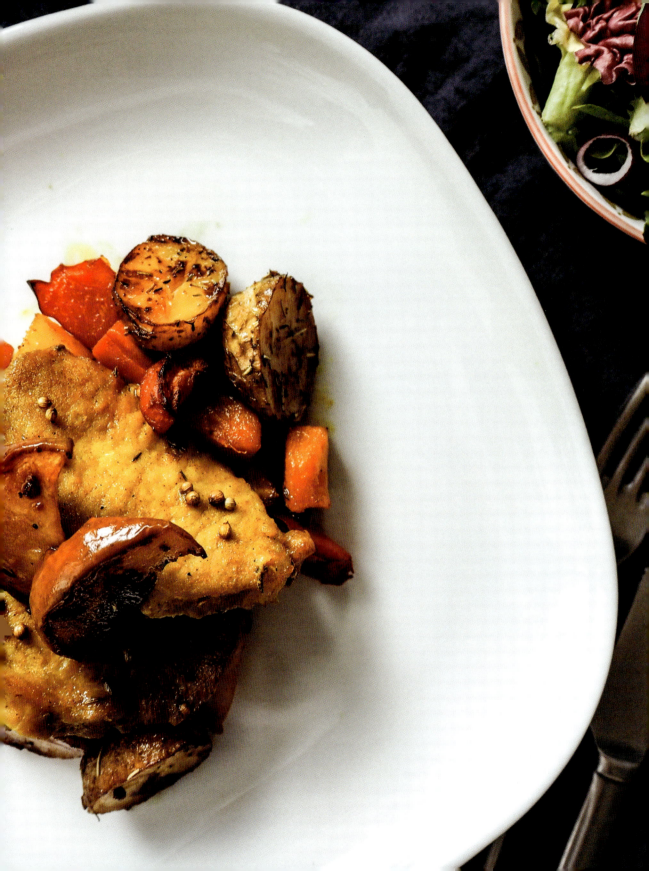

Spiced pork tray bake

🍽 **Serves:** 4 ⏱ **Prep time:** 20 mins 🍲 **Cooking time:** 40 mins

Ingredients

- 6 lean pork chops, fat trimmed off (500g/18oz)
- 16 baby potatoes, chopped in half (600g/1¼lb)
- 4 small parsnips, peeled and cut into chunks
- 4 small carrots, peeled and diced
- 1 red pepper, seeded and chopped
- 1 butternut squash, peeled and cut into chunks
- 3 large red apples, cored and quartered
- 1 tsp. fennel seeds
- 2 tsp. coriander seeds
- 2 garlic cloves, finely chopped
- 1 tsp. ground turmeric
- 3 tbsp. olive oil
- 1 tbsp. honey
- Black pepper

Method

1. Preheat the oven to 190°C/375°F (fan 170°C /325°F) or gas mark 5.

2. Place the pork chops, with fat removed, in a large roasting tin with the potatoes, apples and vegetables.

3. In a ziplock bag crush the fennel and coriander seeds, then mix together the garlic, turmeric, oil, honey and black pepper, and add the crushed seeds.

4. Brush the mixture over the meat and vegetables. Bake in the oven covered with tin foil for 35–40 minutes, turning the vegetables and meat once, until golden brown and tender.

NUTRITION INFORMATION
Amount per serving

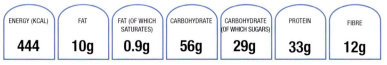

ENERGY (KCAL)	FAT	FAT (OF WHICH SATURATES)	CARBOHYDRATE	CARBOHYDRATE (OF WHICH SUGARS)	PROTEIN	FIBRE
444	10g	0.9g	56g	29g	33g	12g

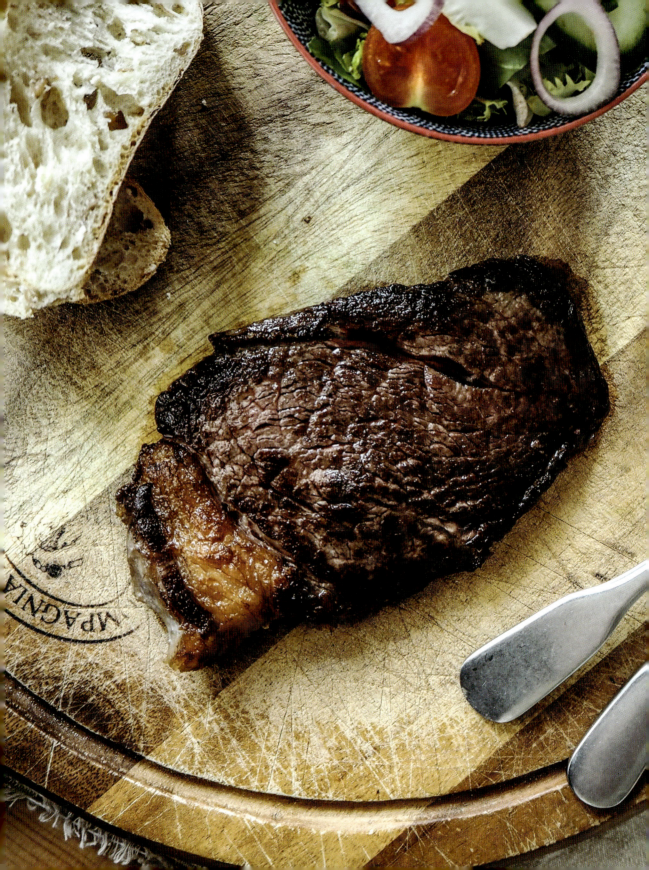

Steak with salsa verde

🍽 **Serves:** 4 ⏱ **Prep time:** 15 mins 🍲 **Cooking time:** 10 mins

Ingredients

- 400g/14oz lean steak (sirloin)
- 1 tbsp. olive oil
- 1 clove garlic, peeled and halved
- Freshly ground black pepper, to taste

For the salsa:
- 1 small bunch fresh coriander
- 1 small bunch fresh mint, leaves only
- 1 clove garlic, peeled and crushed
- 1–2 fresh jalapeno or serrano chillies, deseeded
- 4 large scallions, trimmed
- 2 tomatoes, roughly chopped
- Freshly ground black pepper, to taste
- 1–2 limes, juice of
- 1 tbsp. extra virgin olive oil

Serve with a large green salad and fresh bread or homemade wedges (see page 307).

Method

1. For the salsa verde, chop the coriander (leaves and stalks), mint leaves, garlic, chillies, scallions and tomatoes until fine. Season with pepper and add lime juice and extra virgin olive oil. Mix salsa well.

2. Heat a frying pan or grill pan until very hot and season both sides of the steaks with pepper and a little olive oil.

3. Add the steaks to the pan or grill. Your steaks should take about 6 to 7 minutes per side to cook, depending on how you like them. As it cooks, rub the steak with the cut side of the garlic clove for some extra flavour.

4. Thickly slice the steak and top with the salsa verde. Serve with a large green salad and fresh bread/homemade potato wedges.

NUTRITION INFORMATION
Amount per serving

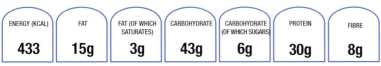

ENERGY (KCAL)	FAT	FAT (OF WHICH SATURATES)	CARBOHYDRATE	CARBOHYDRATE (OF WHICH SUGARS)	PROTEIN	FIBRE
433	15g	3g	43g	6g	30g	8g

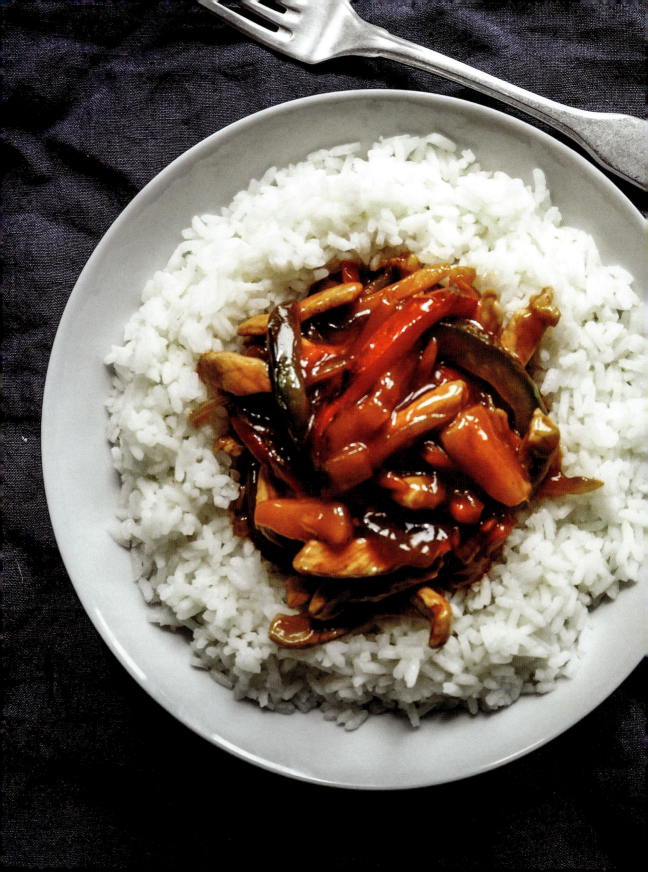

Sweet and sour pork

🍽 **Serves:** 4 ⏱ **Prep time:** 15 mins 🍲 **Cooking time:** 10–15 mins

Ingredients

- 1 x 425g/15oz tin pineapple chunks in juice
- 2 tsp. cornflour
- 1 tbsp. reduced-salt soy sauce
- 2 tbsp. apple cider vinegar
- 1 tbsp. tomato puree
- 1 tsp. five-spice powder
- ½ tsp. dried chilli flakes
- 1 tbsp. sunflower oil
- 1 medium onion, cut into wedges
- 1 green pepper, cut into strips
- 1 red pepper, cut into strips
- 400g/14oz pork pieces
- 2 cloves garlic, crushed
- 2.5cm/1in root ginger, peeled and finely chopped
- Freshly ground black pepper to season

Serve with brown rice.

Method

1. Drain the juice from the pineapple into a bowl.

2. In a separate bowl, mix the cornflour with 1 tbsp. of the pineapple juice to form a paste. Add a further 5 tbsp. of the juice and stir until the paste has dissolved. Add the soy sauce, vinegar, tomato puree, five-spice powder and chilli flakes to the pineapple sauce and mix thoroughly.

3. Warm the oil in a large non-stick frying pan over a medium-high heat. Cook the onion and peppers for 2–3 minutes. Add the pork and cook until browned on all sides.

4. Add the pineapple chunks, garlic, ginger and black pepper to the frying pan, and stir for 1 minute.

5. Mix the sauce and pour into the frying pan. Stir thoroughly, coating all the ingredients in the sauce. Bring to the boil and reduce the temperature. Allow to simmer, stirring occasionally – for about 5 minutes, until the pork is cooked through.

NUTRITION INFORMATION
Amount per serving

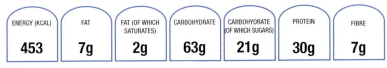

ENERGY (KCAL)	FAT	FAT (OF WHICH SATURATES)	CARBOHYDRATE	CARBOHYDRATE (OF WHICH SUGARS)	PROTEIN	FIBRE
453	7g	2g	63g	21g	30g	7g

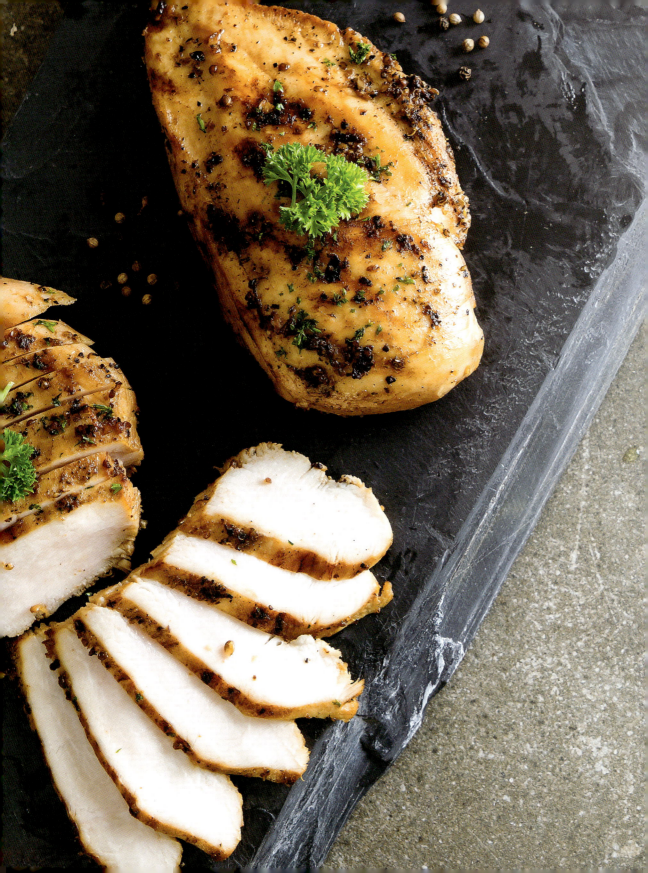

Poultry

Chicken and broccoli bake

Chicken casserole

Chicken goujons

Chicken, bean and kale stew

Chicken stir-fry with cashew nuts

Fruity chicken tagine

Grilled chicken with green lentil dahl

Tandoori chicken fillet burger

Turkey fajitas

Pasta with turkey, almond and rocket

Chicken Lahori

Creamy chicken and tomato bake

Chicken and mushroom risotto

Spicy sweet Thai noodles with chicken

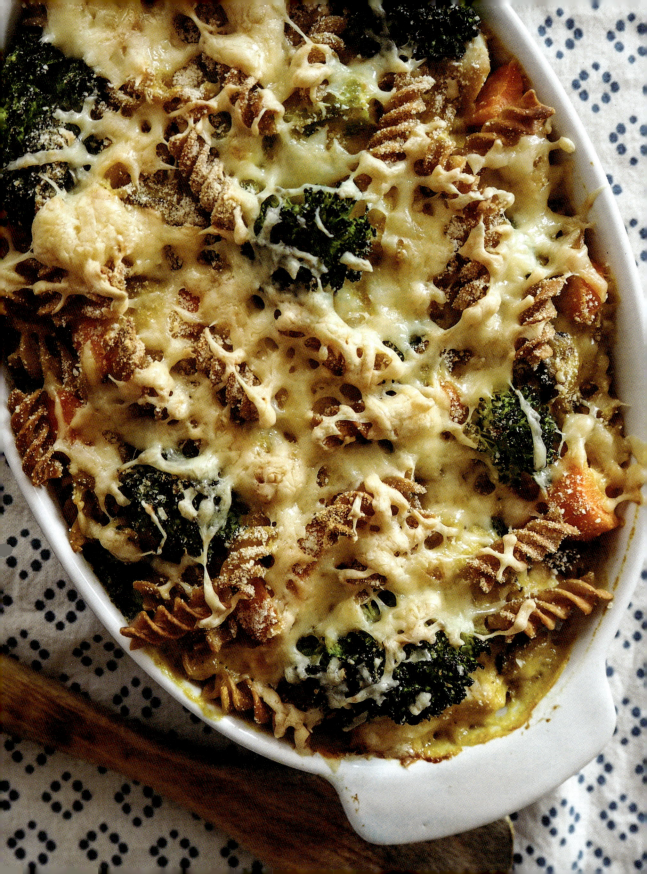

Chicken and broccoli bake

Serves: 4 **Prep time:** 15 mins **Cooking time:** 30 mins

Ingredients

- 250g/2½ cups brown pasta spirals (raw weight)
- 300g/10½oz broccoli, broken up into florets
- 3 medium carrots, peeled and chopped
- 1 tbsp. vegetable oil
- 400g/14oz chicken breasts, diced
- 1 large onion, chopped
- 200g/2½ cups mushrooms, washed and sliced
- 2 cloves garlic, crushed
- Freshly ground black pepper, to season
- 250ml/1 cup low-fat milk
- 150ml/¾ cup chicken stock or homemade chicken stock
- 1 tsp. mustard powder or curry powder
- 3 tsp. cornflour mixed with 2 tsp. water
- 75g/¾ cup fresh wholemeal breadcrumbs
- 50g/½ cup grated low-fat cheese

Method

1. Preheat the oven to 180°C/350°F (fan 160°C/320°F) or gas mark 4.

2. Cook the pasta as per packet instructions.

3. Parboil or steam the broccoli and carrots for 5 minutes.

4. Meanwhile warm the oil in a frying pan set over a medium heat. Add the chicken and cook for a few minutes just to seal it, then add the onion, mushrooms and garlic. Season with a pinch of pepper and cook for about 5 minutes more, until the onion has softened. Add the broccoli and carrots and stir.

5. Add the milk, stock and mustard/curry powder and cook for about 5 minutes.

6. Mix the cornflour with the water in a small bowl, then add to the pan and cook for 1 or 2 minutes, stirring, until creamy and thick.

7. Transfer to an ovenproof baking dish and add the cooked pasta and mix thoroughly. Sprinkle with the breadcrumbs and low-fat grated cheese. Bake in the oven for 10–15 minutes, until the filling is bubbling and the breadcrumbs are golden.

NUTRITION INFORMATION
Amount per serving

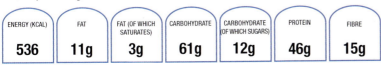

ENERGY (KCAL)	FAT	FAT (OF WHICH SATURATES)	CARBOHYDRATE	CARBOHYDRATE (OF WHICH SUGARS)	PROTEIN	FIBRE
536	11g	3g	61g	12g	46g	15g

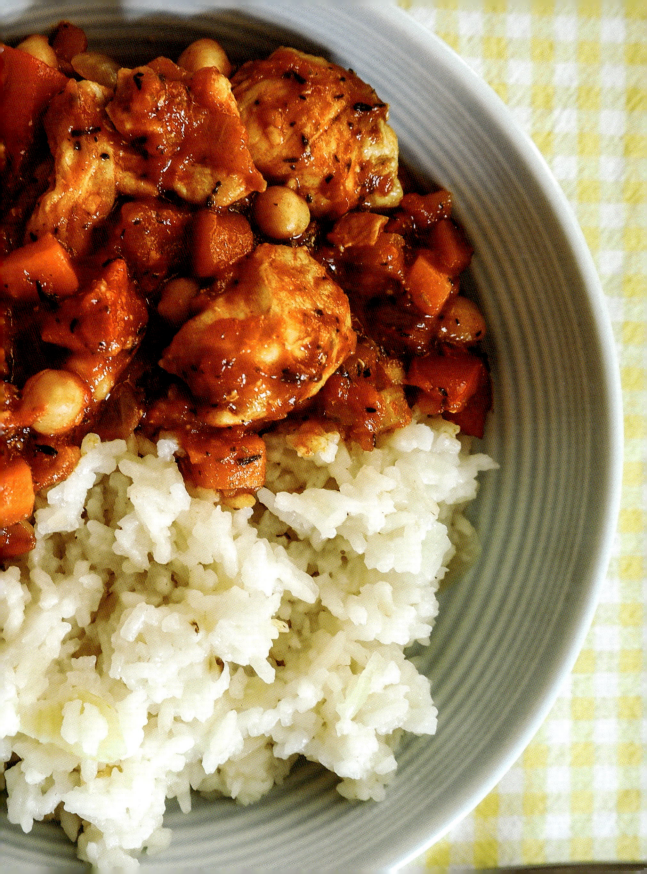

Chicken casserole

🍽 **Serves:** 4 ⏱ **Prep time:** 15 mins 🍲 **Cooking time:** 50 mins

Ingredients

- 1 tbsp. olive oil
- 1 onion, finely chopped
- 4–5 medium carrots, washed and cut into chunks
- 2 medium celery sticks, finely chopped
- 400g/14oz chicken breast, chopped
- 2 garlic cloves, peeled and crushed
- 1 tsp. paprika
- ½ tsp. ground cumin
- 1 tsp. dried thyme
- 2 x 400g/14oz tins chopped tomatoes
- 1 chicken stock cube
- 1 red pepper, diced
- 1 x 400g/14oz tin chickpeas, drained
- 4 tsp. cornflour mixed with 4 tsp. water

Serve with rice or potatoes.

Method

1. Heat the oil in a large heavy-based pan. Add the onion, carrot and celery and cook gently until softened.

2. Add the chicken pieces, garlic, spices and thyme. Cook until the chicken is brown on all sides.

3. Pour in the tomatoes, plus one extra half a tin of water or enough to cover the chicken and vegetables.

4. Crumble in the stock cube and add the red pepper. Bring to a simmer and cook uncovered for 40 minutes.

5. Add the chickpeas and cook for a further five minutes.

6. Stir in the cornflour and water to thicken before serving.

7. Serve with rice or potatoes.

NUTRITION INFORMATION
Amount per serving

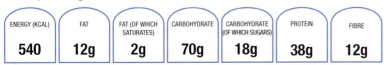

ENERGY (KCAL)	FAT	FAT (OF WHICH SATURATES)	CARBOHYDRATE	CARBOHYDRATE (OF WHICH SUGARS)	PROTEIN	FIBRE
540	12g	2g	70g	18g	38g	12g

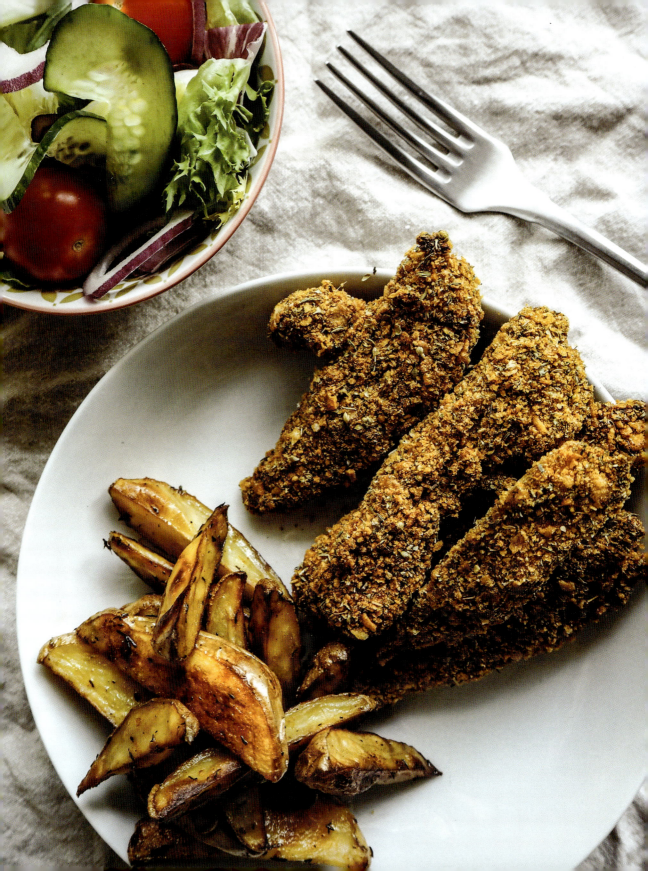

Chicken goujons

Serves: 4 **Prep time:** 15 mins **Cooking time:** 1 hour

Ingredients

- 4 large potatoes, washed, with skin on, and cut into wedges
- 1 tbsp. sunflower oil
- Seasoning of choice, e.g. smoked paprika
- 150g/2 cups cornflakes, crushed
- Pinch of pepper
- 2 tsp. mixed herbs
- 2 eggs, beaten
- 400g/14oz chicken breasts, cut into 1in strips
- Large mixed salad

Method

1. Preheat the oven to 190°C/375°F (fan 170°C /325°F) or gas mark 5.

2. Chop the potatoes into wedges and place in a ziplock bag. Add the oil and seasoning, seal the bag and shake to evenly distribute the oil and seasoning on the wedges.

3. Mix the crushed cornflakes, pepper and mixed herbs together in a bowl.

4. Beat the eggs in a separate bowl.

5. Dip the chicken pieces in the egg and then in the seasoned cornflake crumbs, pressing them on well.

6. Place the coated chicken and potato wedges in a casserole dish lined with greaseproof paper.

7. Bake the wedges in the preheated oven for 30–40 minutes until golden brown and on a separate tray bake the chicken for 20–30 minutes until cooked.

8. Serve with a large side salad.

NUTRITION INFORMATION
Amount per serving

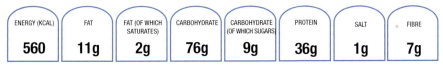

ENERGY (KCAL)	FAT	FAT (OF WHICH SATURATES)	CARBOHYDRATE	CARBOHYDRATE (OF WHICH SUGARS)	PROTEIN	SALT	FIBRE
560	11g	2g	76g	9g	36g	1g	7g

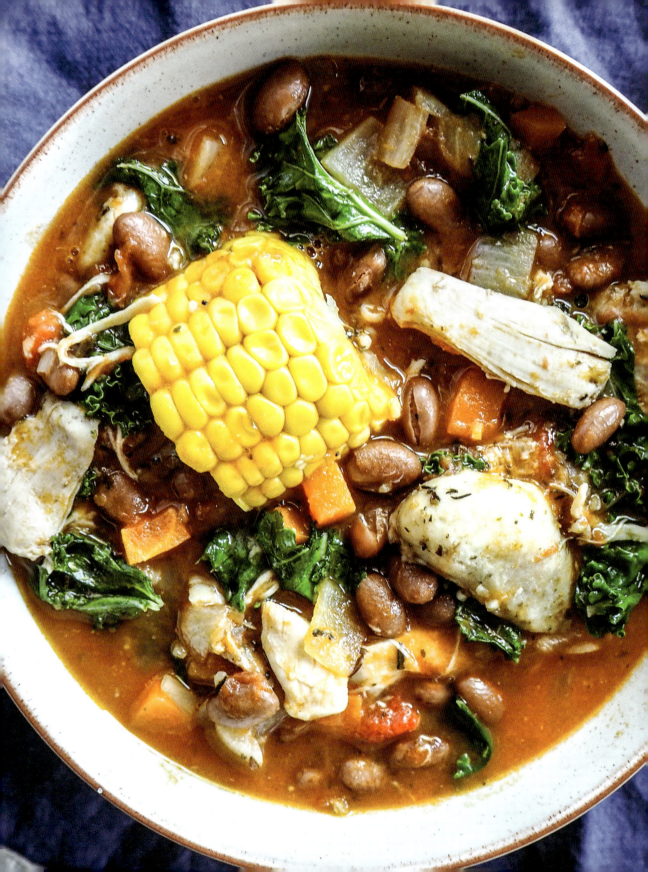

Chicken, bean and kale stew

🍽 **Serves:** 4–6 ⏱ **Prep time:** 10 mins 🍲 **Cooking time:** 35–40 mins

Ingredients

- 1 tbsp. rapeseed oil
- 1 medium onion, chopped
- 2 cloves garlic, crushed
- 1 carrot, diced
- 1 tbsp. ground cumin
- 1 tsp. red chilli flakes (optional)
- 1 tin plum tomatoes, chopped
- 1 tin pinto beans or chickpeas, drained
- 600ml/2½ cups chicken stock
- 4–6 small corn on the cob (can use frozen)
- ¼–½ cooked roast chicken, shredded (~360g/13oz cooked meat)
- 6 large kale leaves, stalks removed and finely chopped
- Black pepper to season

Serve with fresh bread, baked potato, brown pasta or brown rice.

Method

1. Heat the oil in a large saucepan over a medium heat and add the onion, garlic and carrot. Cover with a lid and sweat over a low to medium heat for 10 minutes, stirring occasionally.

2. Remove the lid and turn up the heat slightly. Add the cumin and chilli flakes and cook for 1 minute. Add the chopped tomatoes, beans and stock, and then bring to the boil and add the corn on the cob pieces. Turn down the heat and simmer gently for 15 minutes to cook the corn.

3. Finally add the shredded chicken and chopped kale. Taste and season. Continue to gently simmer for 10–15 minutes. Add more water or stock if it's too thick. Taste to check the seasoning before ladling into warm bowls, with one corn piece per person.

4. Serve with fresh bread, baked potato, brown pasta or brown rice.

NUTRITION INFORMATION
Amount per serving

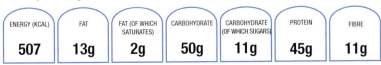

ENERGY (KCAL)	FAT	FAT (OF WHICH SATURATES)	CARBOHYDRATE	CARBOHYDRATE (OF WHICH SUGARS)	PROTEIN	FIBRE
507	13g	2g	50g	11g	45g	11g

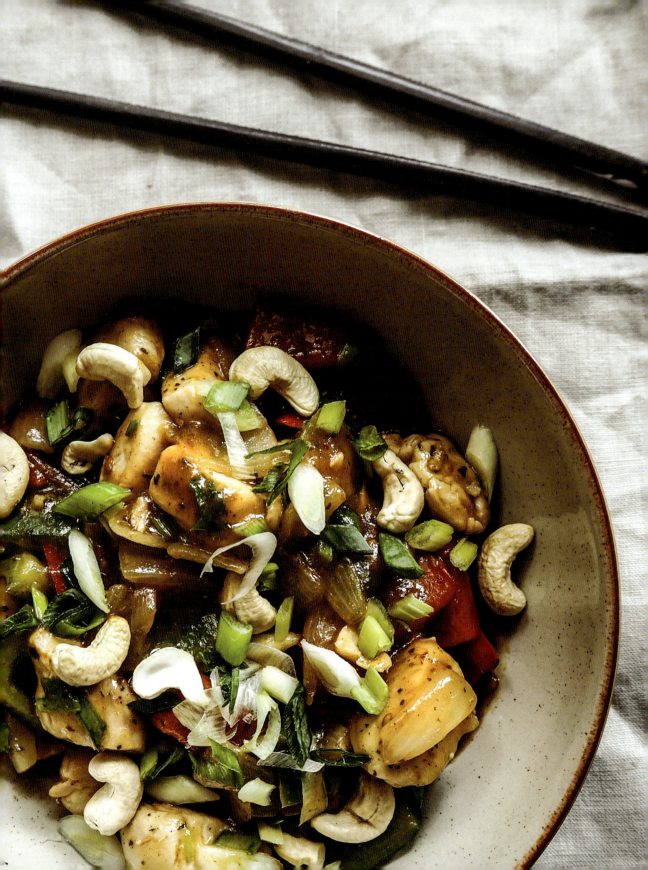

Chicken stir-fry with cashew nuts

🍽 **Serves:** 6 ⏱ **Prep time:** 20 mins 🍲 **Cooking time:** 20 mins (plus time for marinating)

Ingredients

- 4 chicken fillets, cut in to chunks (400g/14oz)
- 60g/⅓ cup unsalted cashew nuts
- 2 tbsp. sunflower oil
- 2 onions, peeled and cut in chunks
- 2 red peppers, washed and cut in chunks
- 2 green peppers, washed and cut in chunks
- 2 cloves garlic, peeled and crushed
- 1 tbsp. ginger, peeled and grated
- 3 spring onions, peeled and sliced
- 1 tbsp. oyster sauce
- 1 tsp. soy sauce
- 100ml/½ cup chicken stock or water
- 2 tsp. cornflour mixed with 2 tbsp. water
- Finely shredded spring onion to garnish

Marinade:
- 2 tsp. cornflour mixed with 2 tbsp. water and 2 tsp. light reduced-sodium soy sauce

Serve with boiled brown rice, 70g/1/3 cup per person.

Method

1. Coat the chicken in the marinade mixture and allow to marinate for minimum 30 minutes.

2. Toast the cashew nuts for 2–3 minutes in a dry, non-stick frying pan, stirring regularly until they are golden brown in colour.

3. Heat half the oil in a wok. Fry the onion, red and green peppers, garlic, ginger and spring onions for about 2 minutes. Remove to a plate.

4. Heat the remaining oil and add the chicken with the marinade. Wait a few seconds before moving, to allow the cornflour coating to set. If you move the chicken straight away it will stick to the wok.

5. Stir-fry the chicken for about 5 minutes. Add the vegetables back into the wok.

6. Turn down the heat and add the oyster sauce, soy sauce and the chicken stock.

7. Add the cornflour mixture and bring to the boil while stirring, until thickened.

8. Finally add the shredded spring onions and the toasted cashew nuts.

9. Serve with boiled wholegrain rice.

NUTRITION INFORMATION
Amount per serving

ENERGY (KCAL)	FAT	FAT (OF WHICH SATURATES)	CARBOHYDRATE	CARBOHYDRATE (OF WHICH SUGARS)	PROTEIN	FIBRE
463	14g	2g	56g	8.4g	26g	6g

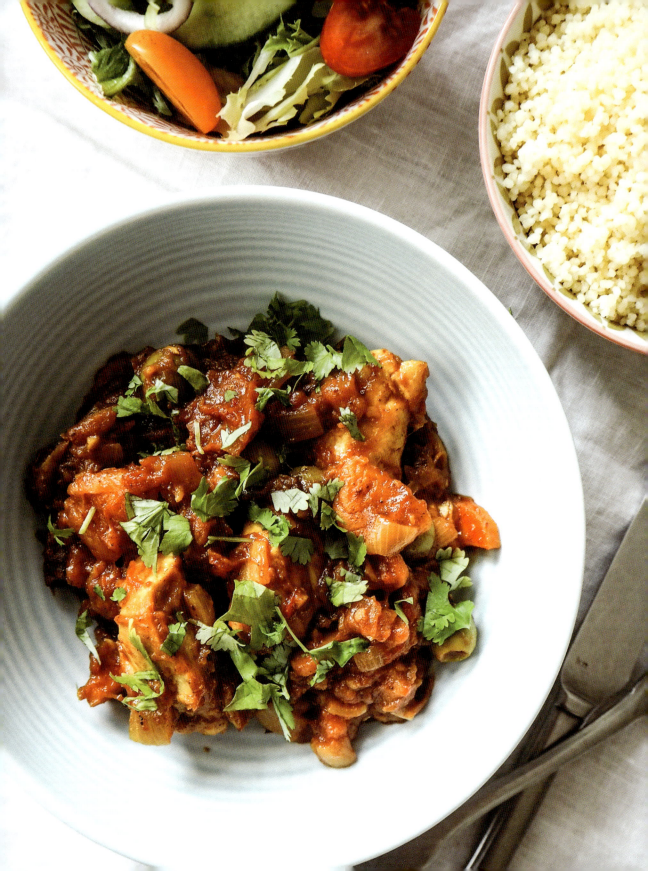

Fruity chicken tagine

🍽 **Serves:** 4 ⏱ **Prep time:** 10 mins 🍲 **Cooking time:** 1 hour

Ingredients

- 2 tbsp. olive or rapeseed oil
- 4 chicken breasts, cut into large cubes (500g/18oz)
- 2 medium onions, chopped
- 2 carrots, chopped
- 2 garlic cloves, chopped
- Thumb-sized piece root ginger, grated, or 1 tsp. ground ginger
- ½ tsp. saffron (optional)
- 2 tsp. ras-el-hanout (North African spice blend) or Moroccan spice mix
- ½ tsp. turmeric
- 1 tsp. ground cinnamon or 2 cinnamon sticks
- 1 tsp. freshly ground pepper
- Small handful chopped coriander
- 100g/½ cup green olives, rinsed
- 50g/¼ cup dates (stones removed) or 50g/¼ cup apricots, halved
- 1 x 400g/14oz tin chopped tomatoes
- 300ml/1¼ cups chicken stock
- 2 tbsp. honey
- Juice of 1 lemon

Serve with cooked couscous or brown rice and large green salad.

Method

1. In a large lidded saucepan, brown the chicken pieces in 1 tbsp. oil. Remove the chicken from the pan and set aside.

2. Add the remaining oil, onions, carrots, garlic and ginger to the pan and sauté until softened. Stir in the spices and half the coriander and cook for 1 minute. Add the olives, dates/apricots and tomatoes, then return the chicken to the pan and stir until the chicken is coated in the spice mix.

3. Add the stock, honey and lemon juice and bring the mixture to the boil. Reduce the heat and simmer for 45 minutes or until the chicken is tender and fully cooked through. Season to taste.

4. Sprinkle with the remaining coriander and serve with couscous or brown rice and green salad.

NUTRITION INFORMATION
Amount per serving

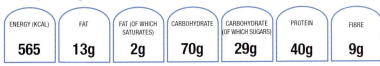

ENERGY (KCAL)	FAT	FAT (OF WHICH SATURATES)	CARBOHYDRATE	CARBOHYDRATE (OF WHICH SUGARS)	PROTEIN	FIBRE
565	13g	2g	70g	29g	40g	9g

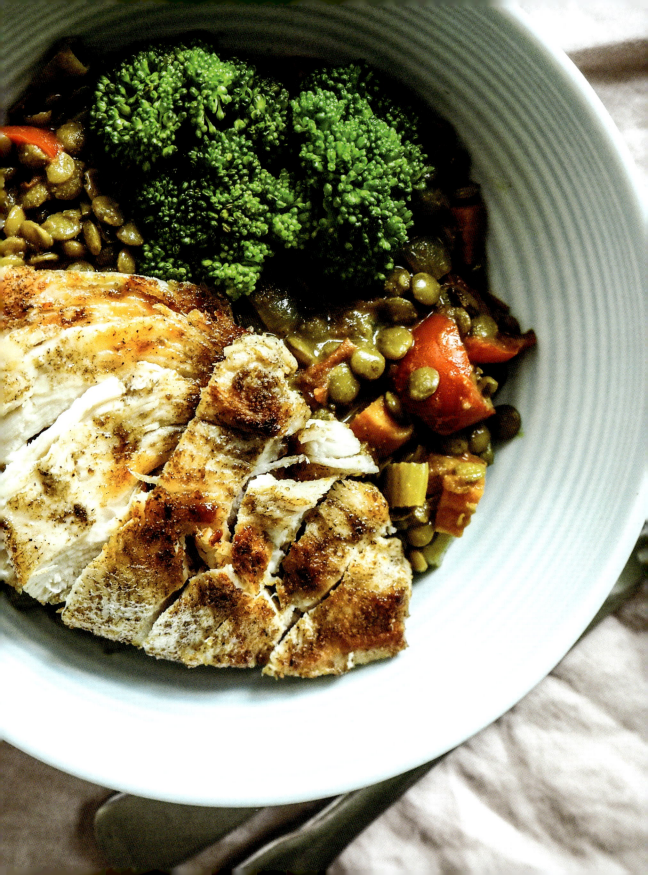

Grilled chicken with green lentil dahl

🍽 **Serves:** 4 ⏱ **Prep time:** 20 mins 🍲 **Cooking time:** 40 mins

Ingredients

- 2 tbsp. vegetable oil
- 1 onion, finely chopped
- 2 garlic cloves, crushed
- 1 thumb-sized piece of ginger, finely chopped/grated
- 1 mild chilli, deseeded and finely chopped
- 1 carrot, chopped
- 1 stick celery, chopped
- 1 red bell pepper, chopped
- 4 plum tomatoes, chopped
- 2 tsp. curry powder
- 2 tsp. cumin
- 1 tsp. turmeric
- 250g/1¼ cups dried green lentils
- 200g/1 cup light coconut milk
- 500ml/2 cups chicken stock
- 1 tsp. black pepper
- 400g/14oz lean chicken breast fillets, grilled
- 400g/14oz broccoli

Method

1. Heat a tbsp. of oil in a pan. Sauté the chopped onion, ginger, chilli and garlic for 5 minutes.

2. Add the chopped celery, carrot, tomatoes and red pepper to the pan and cook for 5 minutes.

3. Add the turmeric, curry powder, ½ tsp. pepper and half of the cumin and cook for 2 minutes.

4. Tip the lentils, stock and half of the coconut milk into the pan. Bring to the boil, then cover and cook for 20–30 minutes over a low heat until the lentils are soft.

5. Meanwhile, prepare the chicken. Mix together 1 tbsp. of oil, ½ tsp. black pepper and 1 tsp. cumin. Trim the fat off the chicken fillets and rub the mixture on them.

6. Heat a grill pan (or normal frying pan) and cook the chicken over a medium heat for 8–10 minutes a side until fully cooked through.

7. Steam the broccoli for ~8 minutes, or boil for ~5 minutes.

8. Finish the dahl by stirring in the rest of the coconut milk and serve with chicken and broccoli.

NUTRITION INFORMATION
Amount per serving

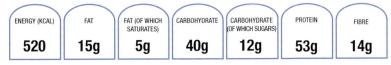

ENERGY (KCAL)	FAT	FAT (OF WHICH SATURATES)	CARBOHYDRATE	CARBOHYDRATE (OF WHICH SUGARS)	PROTEIN	FIBRE
520	15g	5g	40g	12g	53g	14g

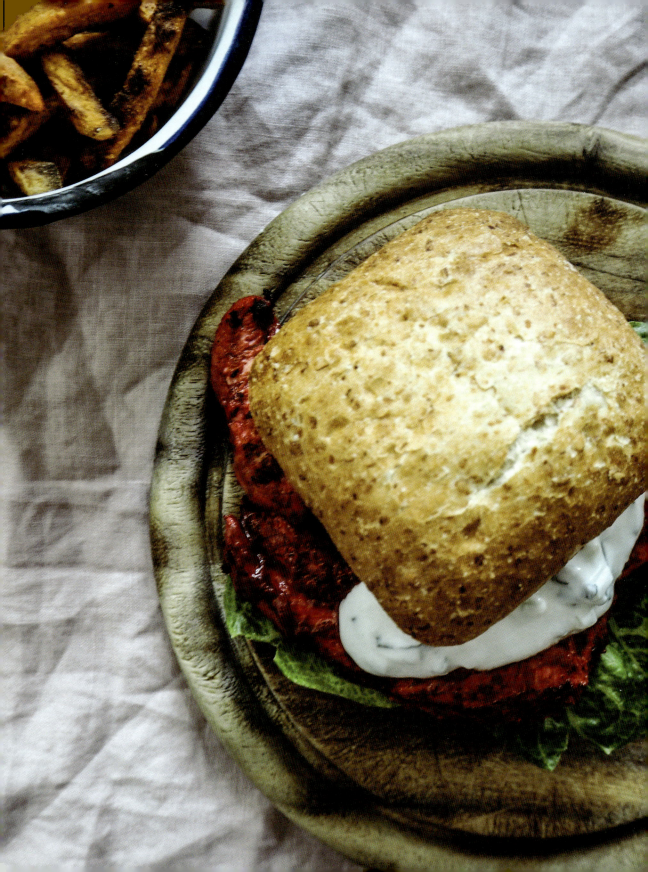

Tandoori chicken fillet burger

🍽 **Serves:** 4 ⏱ **Prep time:** 10 mins 🍲 **Cooking time:** 15–20 mins

Ingredients

- 4 chicken breasts, skinless (400g/14oz)
- 2 tbsp. tandoori paste
- 1 tsp. dried coriander
- 2 tsp. rapeseed oil
- 2 tbsp. natural low-fat yogurt
- A small bunch of fresh mint leaves, finely chopped
- ½ cucumber, diced
- A few lettuce leaves, washed and cut into slices
- 4 wholemeal burger buns, halved and toasted

Serve with large side salad.

Method

1. In a bowl, add the chicken breasts, tandoori paste, coriander and a little oil. Mix together. Toss the chicken breasts in the marinade until the chicken is coated.

2. Heat the rest of the oil in a large frying pan over a medium heat. Cook the chicken breasts for 8–10 minutes each side or until cooked through.

3. In another bowl, combine the yogurt, mint and cucumber.

4. Assemble your burger with lettuce on the base of the bun, top with the chicken burger and a dollop of the mint and cucumber yogurt. Top with the other half of the bun and serve with a large side salad.

NUTRITION INFORMATION
Amount per serving

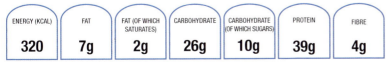

ENERGY (KCAL)	FAT	FAT (OF WHICH SATURATES)	CARBOHYDRATE	CARBOHYDRATE (OF WHICH SUGARS)	PROTEIN	FIBRE
320	7g	2g	26g	10g	39g	4g

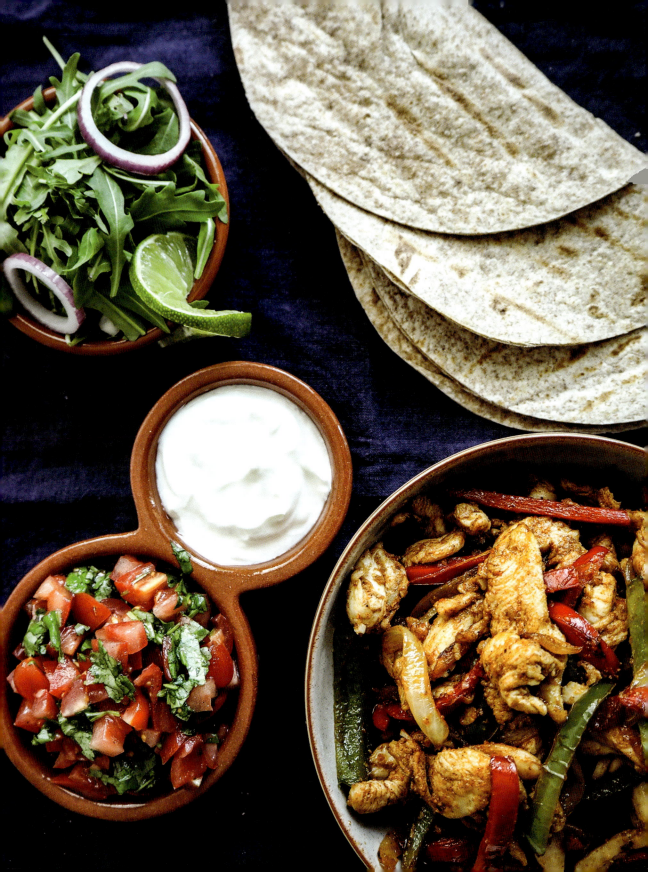

Turkey fajitas

🍽 **Serves:** 4 ⏱ **Prep time:** 30 mins (plus time for marinating) 🍲 **Cooking time:** 15 mins

Ingredients

- 400g/14oz lean turkey breast, cut into strips
- 2 red peppers and 2 green peppers, cut into strips
- 2 onions, cut into strips

Marinade:
- 2 cloves of garlic, crushed
- 1 tbsp. olive oil
- 1 tbsp. smoked paprika
- 1 tbsp. ground coriander
- 1 tsp. cumin
- Pinch of cracked black pepper
- Juice of 1 lime
- 3–4 drops of Tabasco (if desired)

Salsa:
- 225g/1 cup of cherry tomatoes, chopped
- 1 small red onion, peeled and finely chopped
- 1 red chilli (or half a chilli, depending on the level of heat desired)
- 1 handful of coriander, roughly chopped
- Juice of 1 lime

To serve:
- 100ml/½ cup low-fat natural yogurt
- Mixed green salad
- 6 large or 12 small wholegrain soft tortilla wraps

Method

1. Preheat the oven to 200°C/400°F (fan 180°C/350°F) or gas mark 6 and wrap the tortillas in foil.

2. Add the turkey, onion and peppers to a mixing bowl with the marinade ingredients.

3. Heat a griddle pan until hot and add the turkey, vegetable and marinade mixture. Keep them moving over a high heat using tongs so you get a charring effect and until the turkey is fully cooked.

4. Put the tortillas in the oven wrapped in the foil and heat for roughly 8 minutes.

5. To make the salsa, chop the ingredients and combine.

6. Once the turkey is cooked through, tip the pan contents into a large bowl and serve with the heated tortillas, green salad, natural yogurt and homemade salsa.

NUTRITION INFORMATION
Amount per serving

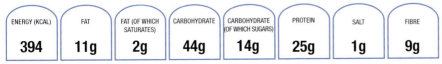

ENERGY (KCAL)	FAT	FAT (OF WHICH SATURATES)	CARBOHYDRATE	CARBOHYDRATE (OF WHICH SUGARS)	PROTEIN	SALT	FIBRE
394	11g	2g	44g	14g	25g	1g	9g

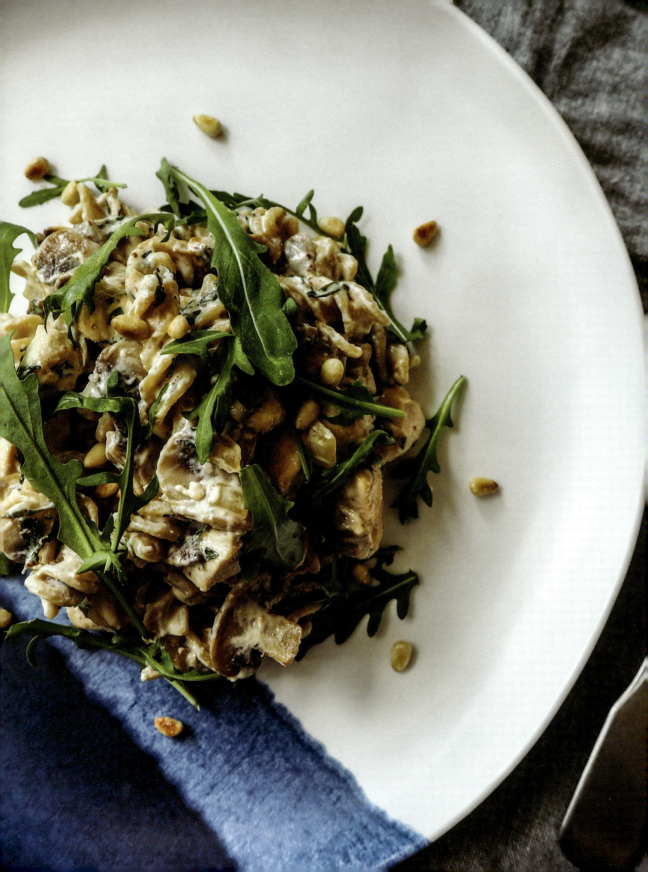

Pasta with turkey, almond and rocket

🍽 **Serves:** 4 ⏱ **Prep time:** 15 mins 🍲 **Cooking time:** 20 mins

Ingredients

- 280g/2¾ cups of wholewheat pasta
- 3 tbsp. almonds
- 1 tbsp. of olive oil
- 200g/2½ cups of mushrooms, washed and sliced
- 1 onion, thinly sliced (150g/5oz)
- 2 garlic cloves, crushed
- 1 tsp. of fresh thyme leaves – or ½ tsp. of dried thyme
- 300g/11oz of turkey, cubed
- 2 tsp. of wholegrain mustard
- 100ml/½ cup of low-fat crème fraiche
- 120g/4oz of rocket, roughly chopped
- 1 tbsp. of fresh basil, chopped

Method

1. Cook the pasta according to pack instructions.

2. Heat a dry frying pan over a medium heat and add the almonds. Gently cook for a few minutes until lightly toasted, tossing occasionally to prevent them from burning. Tip into a bowl and set aside.

3. Add ½ tbsp. of oil to the frying pan and sauté the mushrooms, onion, garlic and thyme for 2 to 3 minutes until softened and just beginning to colour. Remove from the pan.

4. Heat the remaining oil and add the raw turkey and cook, stirring frequently, until cooked through. Return the vegetables to the pan and stir in the mustard and crème fraiche and then bring to a gentle simmer. Cook for 1 minute to heat through but don't allow the mixture to boil.

5. Add the cooked pasta, rocket and basil to the turkey in the pan and mix well. Toss lightly together to combine and season to taste.

6. To serve, spoon the pasta on to warmed serving plates and then sprinkle over the toasted almonds.

NUTRITION INFORMATION
Amount per serving

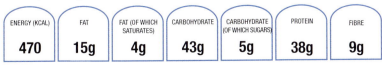

ENERGY (KCAL)	FAT	FAT (OF WHICH SATURATES)	CARBOHYDRATE	CARBOHYDRATE (OF WHICH SUGARS)	PROTEIN	FIBRE
470	15g	4g	43g	5g	38g	9g

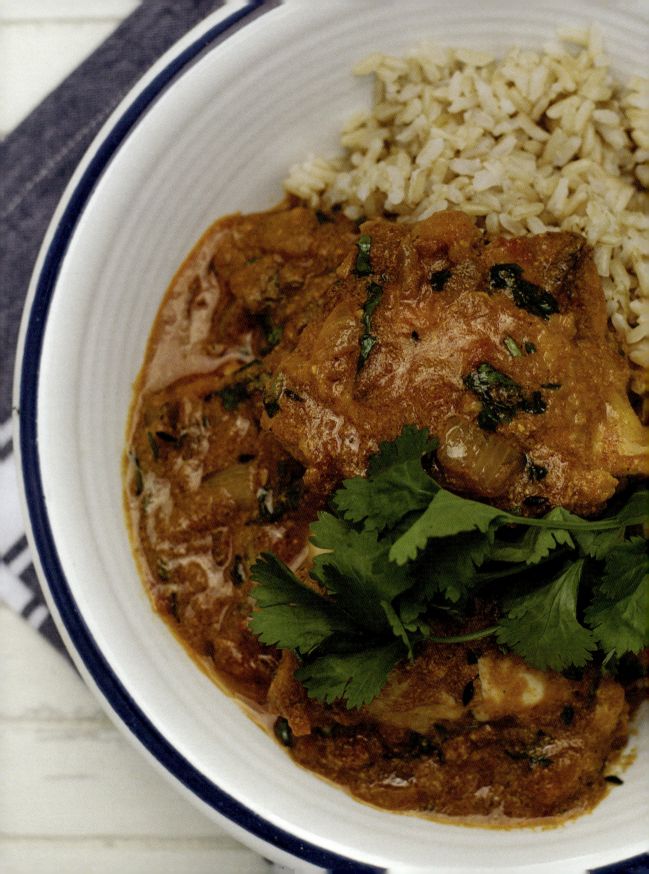

Chicken Lahori

🍽 **Serves:** 4 ⏱ **Prep time:** 25 mins 🍲 **Cooking time:** 40–45 mins

Ingredients

- 2 tbsp. vegetable oil
- 2 black cardamom pods
- 4 green cardamom pods
- 1 tsp. cumin seeds
- 2 bay leaves
- 4 onions, peeled and roughly chopped
- 3 cloves of garlic, peeled and finely chopped
- 3 slices fresh ginger, peeled and finely chopped
- 3 tsp. red chilli powder
- 1½ tbsp. ground coriander
- ½ tsp. ground turmeric
- 4–8 green finger chillies, chopped (depending on desired level of heat)
- 5–6 tomatoes, chopped
- 8 skinless chicken thighs
- 2 tbsp. natural yogurt
- 500ml/2 cups chicken stock or water
- Handful fresh coriander leaves
- 1 tsp. garam masala

Serve with steamed or boiled brown rice.

Method

1. Heat the oil in a large pan or wok and sauté the whole spices and bay leaves until they crackle and pop.

2. Add the onions and cook for 15 minutes over a low heat until lightly browned, then add garlic and ginger and cook for 1 minute.

3. Add the red chilli powder, ground coriander, ground turmeric, green chillies and tomatoes and cook for another 5 minutes.

4. Add the chicken, yogurt and stock. Simmer for 20–25 minutes until the chicken is cooked through. Stir in coriander and garam masala and serve with rice.

NUTRITION INFORMATION
Amount per serving

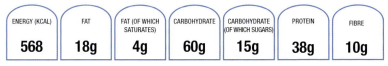

ENERGY (KCAL)	FAT	FAT (OF WHICH SATURATES)	CARBOHYDRATE	CARBOHYDRATE (OF WHICH SUGARS)	PROTEIN	FIBRE
568	18g	4g	60g	15g	38g	10g

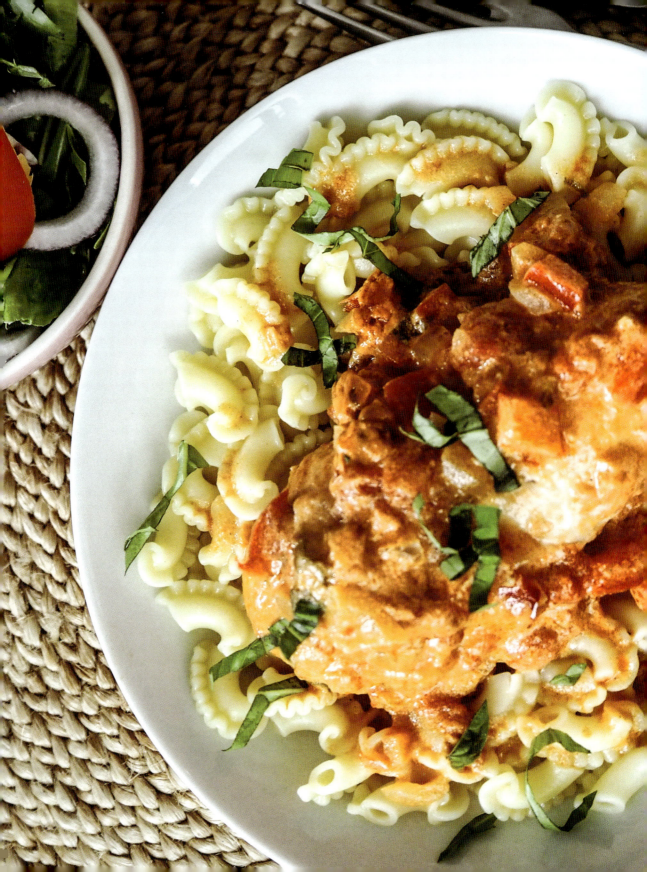

Creamy chicken and tomato bake

🍽 **Serves:** 4 ⏱ **Prep time:** 10 mins 🍲 **Cooking time:** 35–45 mins

Ingredients

- 2 tbsp. olive oil
- 1 onion, finely chopped
- 2 garlic cloves, crushed
- 1 x 400g/14oz tin cherry tomatoes
- Freshly ground black pepper
- 1 tsp. sugar
- 4 tbsp. half-fat crème fraiche (or yogurt)
- Fresh basil (fistful)
- 4 chicken breasts (400g/14oz)
- Serve with short pasta, brown rice or potatoes roasted with olive oil and rosemary and green salad
- Brown rice (raw): 70g/$\frac{1}{3}$ cup per person

Method

1. Fry the onion in the olive oil until softened but not coloured.

2. Add the garlic, tomatoes, pepper and sugar, then simmer for 10–15 minutes.

3. Take off the heat and stir in the crème fraiche and half of the fresh basil, roughly torn.

4. Place the chicken in a baking dish and pour over the sauce.

5. Cook at 190°C/375°F (fan 170°C /325°F) or gas mark 5 for 25–30 minutes or until the chicken is cooked through.

6. Scatter over the remaining basil.

7. Serve with brown rice, wholegrain pasta or potatoes roasted with olive oil and rosemary.

NUTRITION INFORMATION
Amount per serving

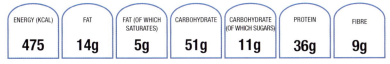

ENERGY (KCAL)	FAT	FAT (OF WHICH SATURATES)	CARBOHYDRATE	CARBOHYDRATE (OF WHICH SUGARS)	PROTEIN	FIBRE
475	14g	5g	51g	11g	36g	9g

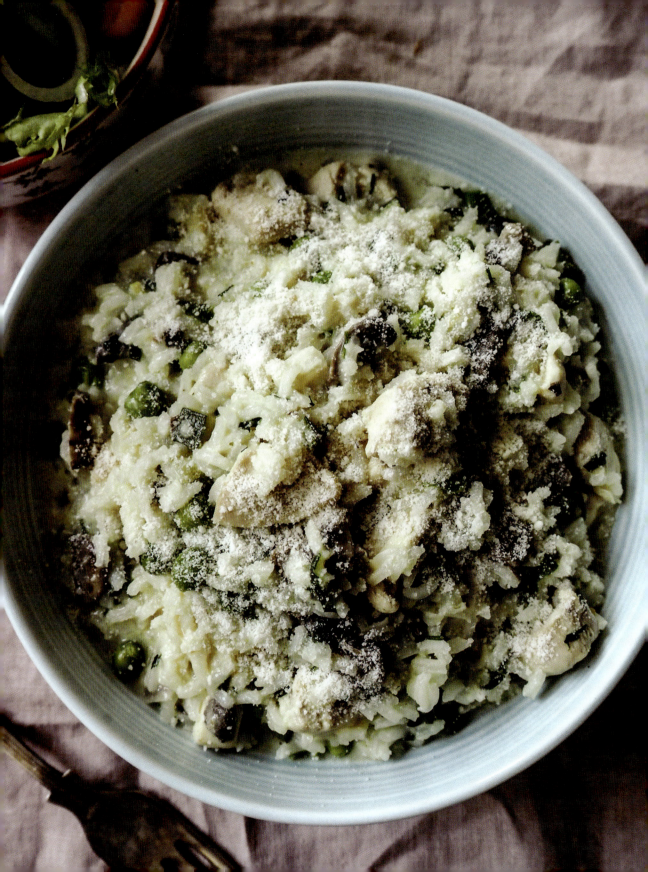

Chicken and mushroom risotto

🍽 **Serves:** 2 ⏱ **Prep time:** 10 mins 🍲 **Cooking time:** 25 mins

Ingredient

- Olive oil spray
- 1 red onion, finely chopped
- 2 chicken breasts, cubed
- ½ courgette, diced
- 150g/2 cups mushrooms, washed and sliced
- 600ml/2½ cups chicken stock
- 100g/½ cup arborio rice
- ½ tsp. ground black pepper (3g/0.1oz)
- 1 tsp. parsley, finely chopped (5g/0.2oz)
- 1 heaped tbsp. low-fat crème fraiche (30g/1oz)
- Garden peas (60g/½ cup)
- 20g/¾oz parmesan, grated
- Green salad to serve

Method

1. Spray a non-stick frying pan or wok with olive oil and cook the onion for 5 minutes until softened.

2. Add the chicken, courgettes and mushrooms and sauté, stirring occasionally, for 10 minutes until the chicken is cooked through. Add a splash of water if the chicken starts to stick to the pan.

3. Meanwhile fill a saucepan with the stock and bring to a gentle simmer. Add the rice to the chicken pan and stir through to make sure it is coated with the chicken and vegetables. Fry for a further 2 minutes.

4. Pour a ladleful of stock into the chicken and rice pan and stir until it is absorbed. This should soak in very quickly. Add another ladleful and stir until absorbed again. Continue in this way until all the stock has been absorbed into the rice.

5. Taste the risotto; it should be soft on the outside but with a slight bite in the middle. If it is too hard, continue to cook, adding a little warm water to keep the consistency creamy. Add the garden peas.

6. Add the parsley, crème fraiche, parmesan and seasoning and stir.

7. Serve immediately with a fresh green salad.

NUTRITION INFORMATION
Amount per serving

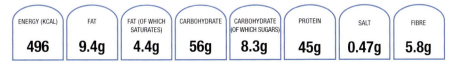

ENERGY (KCAL)	FAT	FAT (OF WHICH SATURATES)	CARBOHYDRATE	CARBOHYDRATE (OF WHICH SUGARS)	PROTEIN	SALT	FIBRE
496	9.4g	4.4g	56g	8.3g	45g	0.47g	5.8g

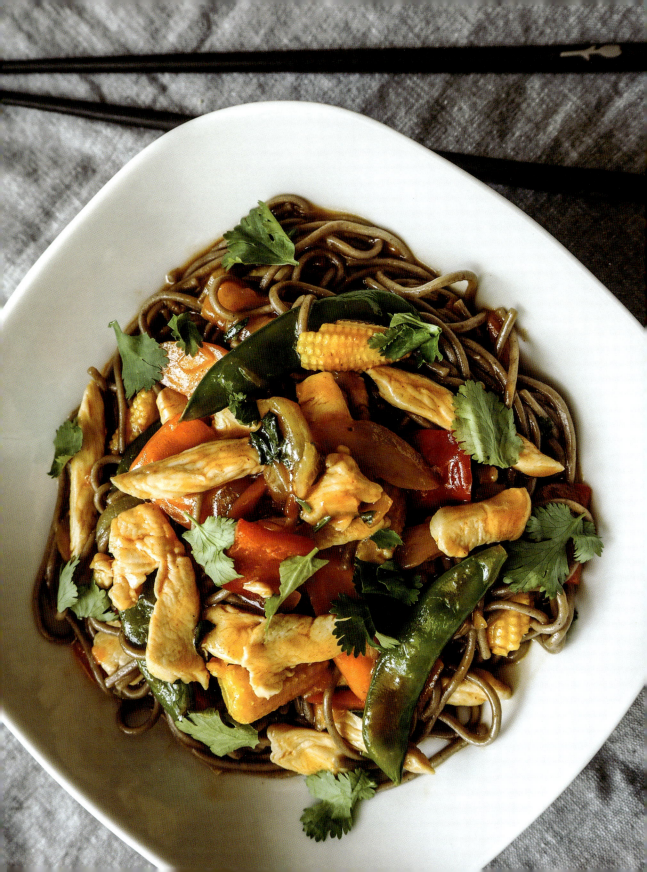

Spicy sweet Thai noodles with chicken

🍽 **Serves:** 2 ⏱ **Prep time:** 10 mins 🍲 **Cooking time:** 10 mins

Ingredients

- 150g/²/₃ cup water
- 2 tbsp. Thai sweet chilli sauce
- 2 tsp. cornflour
- 2 tsp. light soy sauce
- 1 tsp. olive oil
- 1cm/½in piece of ginger, peeled and finely chopped
- 1 clove garlic, peeled and crushed
- 1 red chilli, deseeded and finely chopped
- 2 chicken breasts, cut into small strips
- 150g/5oz mangetout
- 1 red pepper, deseeded and cut into bite-sized pieces
- 200g/7oz baby sweetcorn, cut diagonally
- 2 medium carrots, peeled and chopped into bite-sized pieces
- 2 nests wholewheat noodles
- 1 tbsp. chopped coriander
- A squeeze of lime

Method

1. Mix the water, sweet chilli sauce, cornflour and soy sauce in a jug. Stir well and set aside.

2. Add the olive oil to a medium wok and heat over a high flame. Add the ginger, garlic and chilli. Stir-fry for 1 minute until they release their aroma. Add the chicken and stir-fry until opaque. Then add all the prepared vegetables and continue to stir-fry for a further 3 to 4 minutes.

3. Cook the noodles according to the packet instructions.

4. Drain the noodles once cooked, add them to the wok and mix all the ingredients together. Add the sweet chilli and water mixture and bring the sauce to the boil, stirring until it starts to thicken. When the sauce is thickened, turn off the heat and serve with chopped coriander. Finish with a squeeze of lime.

NUTRITION INFORMATION
Amount per serving

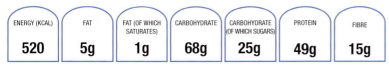

ENERGY (KCAL)	FAT	FAT (OF WHICH SATURATES)	CARBOHYDRATE	CARBOHYDRATE (OF WHICH SUGARS)	PROTEIN	FIBRE
520	5g	1g	68g	25g	49g	15g

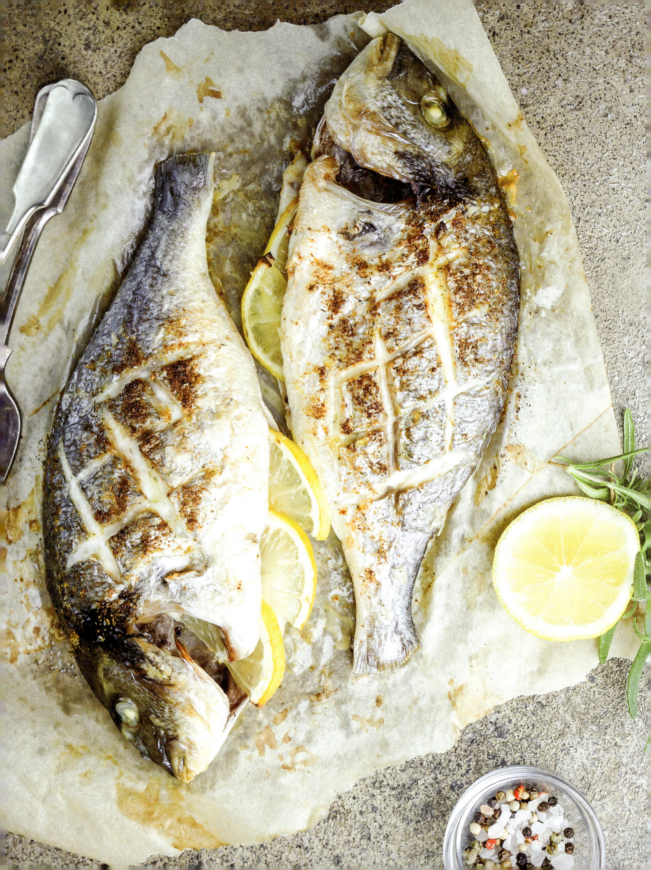

Fish

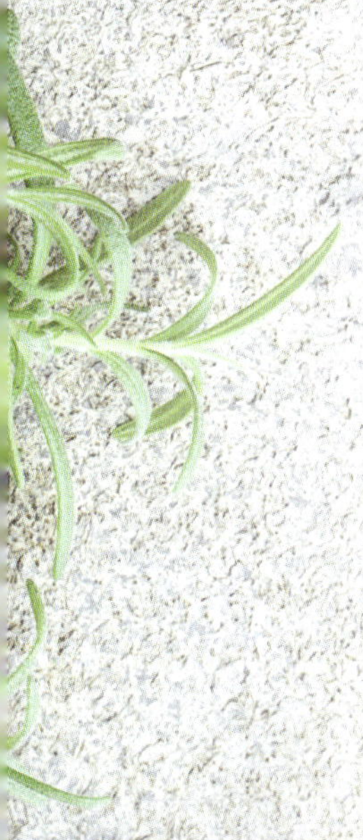

Baked cod with a vine tomato topping

Fish pie

Fish cakes

Fisherman's stew

Glazed salmon

Grilled lemon-scented salmon with chickpea, tomato
and spinach ragout

Healthy fish and chips

Mediterranean fish tray bake

Prawn paella

Salmon linguine

Seared haddock with horseradish aioli

Pasta with mackerel and Mediterranean vegetables

Baked hake/cod with a herb crust

Spicy Italian cod

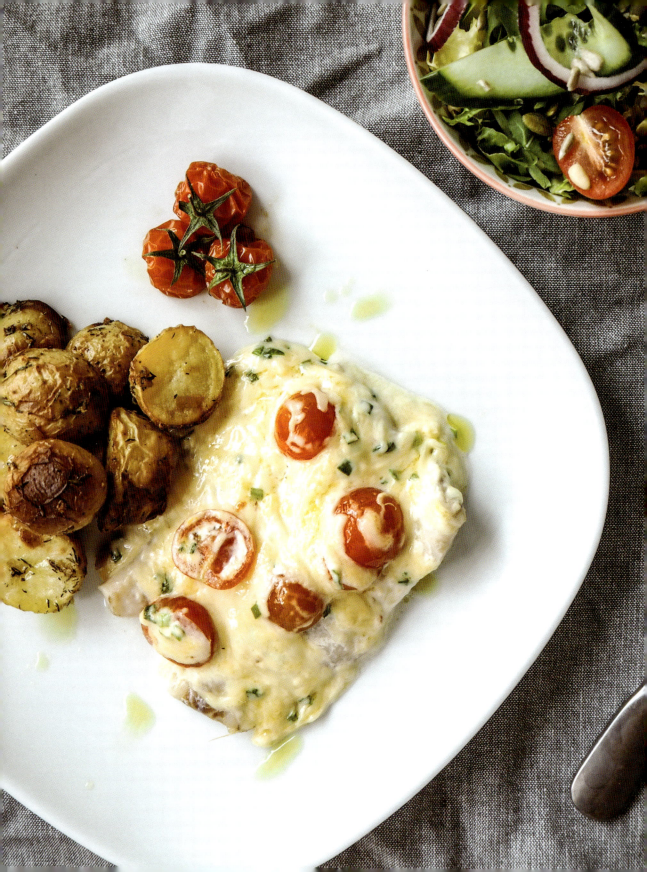

Baked cod with a vine tomato topping

🍽 **Serves:** 4 ⏱ **Prep time:** 5 mins 🍲 **Cooking time:** 20–25 mins

Ingredients

- 200g/1 cup vine/cherry tomatoes, halved
- 120g/1 cup low-fat cheddar cheese, grated
- 40g/3 tbsp. low-fat mayonnaise
- 2 spring onions, chopped
- Black pepper and lemon to season
- 500g/18oz raw cod fillets
- Serve with a portion of salad (150g/5oz) and baked potato/roast garlic baby potatoes (125g/4oz) (see page 305)

Method

1. In a bowl mix the tomatoes, grated cheese, spring onions and mayonnaise. Season with black pepper and a squeeze of lemon.

2. Spread a portion of the mixture on top of each of the cod fillets and wrap in tinfoil.

3. Bake in a preheated oven at 180°C/350°F (fan 160°C/320°F) or gas mark 4 for 15–20 minutes until the fish is cooked through.

4. Serve with a green side salad and a baked potato or roast garlic baby potatoes.

NUTRITION INFORMATION
Amount per serving

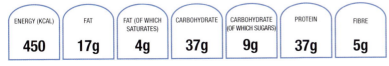

ENERGY (KCAL)	FAT	FAT (OF WHICH SATURATES)	CARBOHYDRATE	CARBOHYDRATE (OF WHICH SUGARS)	PROTEIN	FIBRE
450	17g	4g	37g	9g	37g	5g

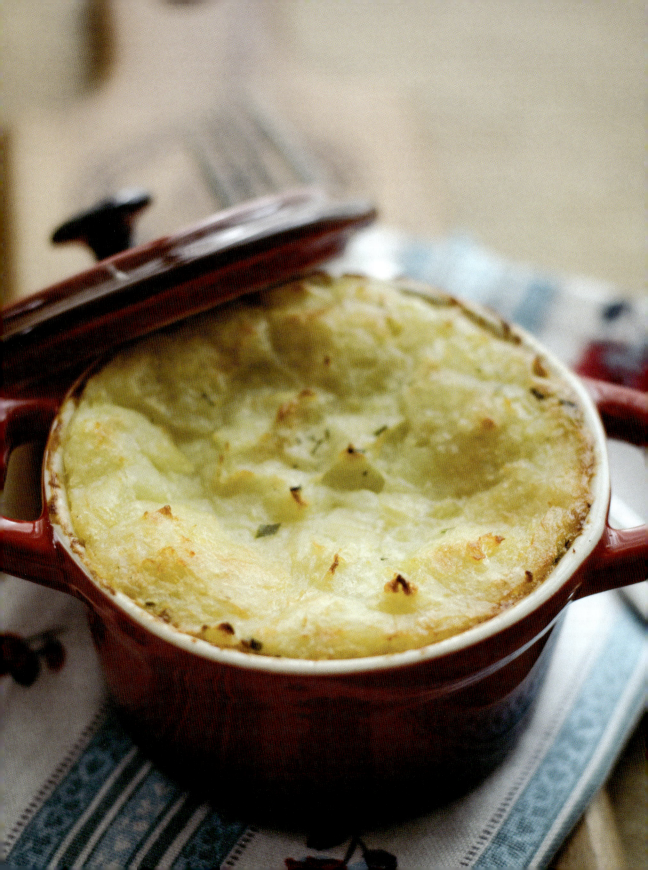

Fish pie

🍽 **Serves:** 4–6 ⏱ **Prep time:** 20 mins 🍲 **Cooking time:** 20 mins

Ingredients

- Juice and zest of half lemon
- Small bunch of fresh parsley
- 150g/5oz raw salmon fillets, skin removed and cut in chunks
- 530g/19oz raw white fish fillets (hake, haddock or cod), skin removed and cut in chunks
- Freshly ground black pepper
- 1 tsp. olive oil
- 1 small onion, peeled and finely chopped
- 1 clove garlic, crushed
- 1 tsp. sugar
- 450g/1lb ripe juicy tomatoes, skinned and chopped (retaining juices), and chopped fresh herbs to taste OR
- 1 x 400g/14oz tin chopped tomatoes with herbs

Topping:
- Champ mash recipe – 800g/28oz (see page 301)
- 2 tbsp. grated low-fat cheese

Serve with green vegetables or a large side salad.

Method

1. Squeeze the lemon juice, reserving the zest; strip and chop the parsley, keeping the stalks.

2. Put the fish into a shallow dish with the lemon zest, parsley stalks and some black pepper; cover with film and microwave until it is just turning opaque. Strain the fish, reserving any cooking juices.

3. Soften the onion and garlic by cooking gently in a little oil over a low heat, then add the chopped tomatoes (with their juices), sugar, chopped parsley and lemon juice to taste.

4. Add the flaked fish and its cooking juices to the tomato mixture, then season to taste with freshly ground black pepper and put into a lightly greased pie dish or shallow casserole.

5. After preparing the champ mash (see page 301), spread it over the fish mixture in the pie dish.

6. Sprinkle with grated cheese and put into a preheated oven, 190°C/375°F (fan 170°C /325°F) or gas mark 5, for about 20 minutes until thoroughly heated and golden brown on top.

7. Serve with plenty of seasonal green vegetables, or a crisp green salad.

NUTRITION INFORMATION
Amount per serving

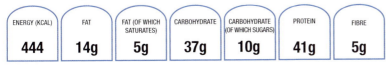

ENERGY (KCAL)	FAT	FAT (OF WHICH SATURATES)	CARBOHYDRATE	CARBOHYDRATE (OF WHICH SUGARS)	PROTEIN	FIBRE
444	14g	5g	37g	10g	41g	5g

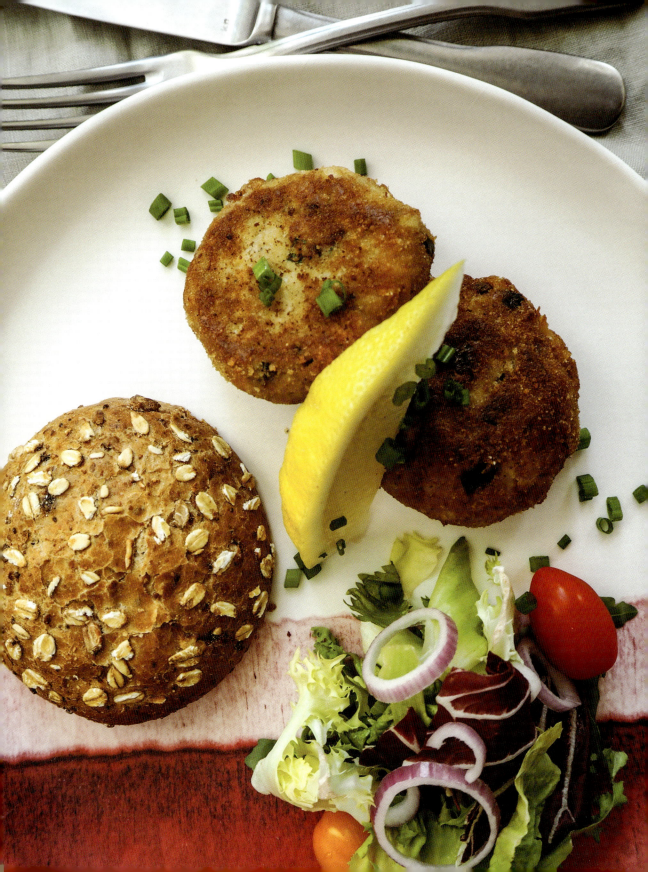

Fish cakes

🍽 **Serves:** 6 (make 12 small fish cakes and serve 2 per person with large salad)

⏱ **Prep time:** 20 mins 🍲 **Cooking time:** 30 mins

Ingredients

- 200g/7oz cod fillet
- 200g/7oz salmon fillet
- 500g/18oz potatoes, boiled
- 100ml/½ cup milk
- 25g/2 tbsp. butter
- 50g/½ cup spring onions, finely chopped

Coating:
- 100g/¾ cup plain flour
- Freshly ground black pepper
- 2 eggs
- 30ml/2 tbsp. milk
- 175g/2 cups breadcrumbs approximately

Serve with dressed green salad and a crusty brown roll/baby potatoes (see page 305) or baked potato wedges (see page 307).

Method

1. Steam the fish until cooked. Remove all skin, ensuring there are no bones, and flake fish.

2. Boil the potatoes and mash, when cooked, with warm milk.

3. Cook the spring onions in the butter until softened.

4. Mix all the ingredients together, season and shape into fish cakes.

5. Whisk the eggs with the milk and season with pepper.

6. Coat each fishcake in flour, then in egg mixture and then in breadcrumbs.

7. Pan-fry until golden brown or bake in the oven until heated through.

8. Serve with a dressed green salad and a crusty brown roll/baby potatoes or baked potato wedges.

NUTRITION INFORMATION
Amount per serving

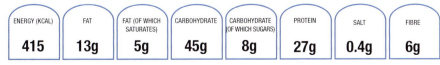

ENERGY (KCAL)	FAT	FAT (OF WHICH SATURATES)	CARBOHYDRATE	CARBOHYDRATE (OF WHICH SUGARS)	PROTEIN	SALT	FIBRE
415	13g	5g	45g	8g	27g	0.4g	6g

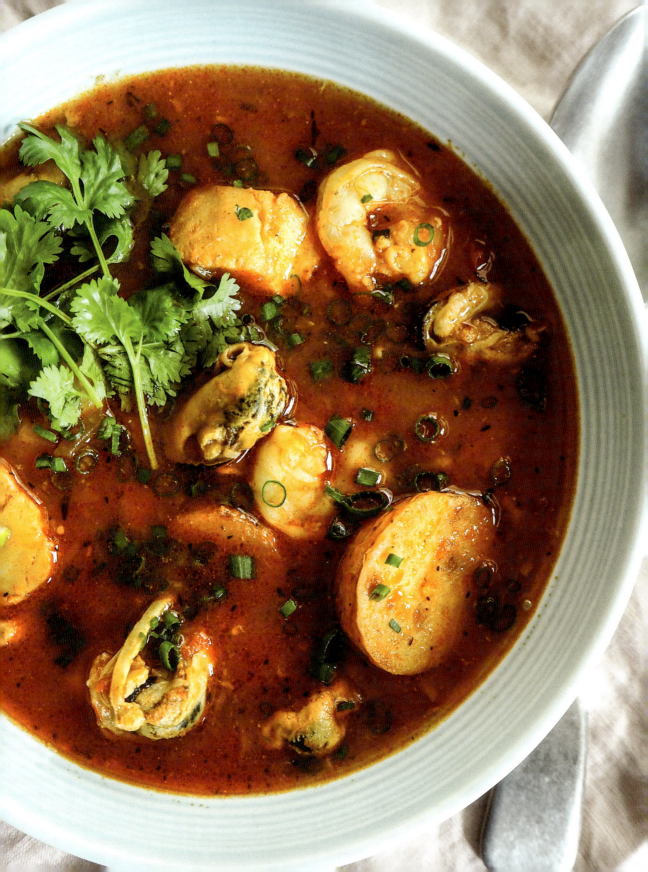

Fisherman's stew

🍽 **Serves:** 4–6 ⏱ **Prep time:** 15 mins 🍲 **Cooking time:** 30 mins

Ingredients

- 1 tbsp. olive oil
- 1 large onion, chopped
- 4 garlic cloves, chopped
- 1 tsp. paprika
- 2 chillies, finely chopped
- 1 tsp. ground cumin
- 550ml/2$^1/_3$ cups chicken stock
- 400g/14oz tin chopped tomatoes
- 200g/7oz large peeled raw prawns
- 300g/11oz halibut or other firm white fish fillets, cut into 2½cm/1in pieces
- 300g/11oz cleaned mussels (discard any with broken shells)
- 800g/28oz small new potatoes, halved and boiled
- Juice 1 lime

Serve with green salad or steamed green vegetables.

Method

1. Heat the olive oil in a large saucepan over a medium heat. Add the onion and garlic, season and cook for about 5 minutes or until softened.

2. Add the paprika, chopped chillies, cumin and tomatoes. Simmer for 5 minutes, add the stock then puree until very fine in a blender.

3. Pour back into the pan and bring to the boil. Reduce the heat and simmer for 10 minutes. When close to eating, add the prawns, fish pieces, mussels and potatoes. Place a lid on top and cook for 8–10 minutes over a medium heat. Discard any mussels that remain closed. Add the lime juice.

4. Serve with a green salad or steamed green vegetables.

NUTRITION INFORMATION
Amount per serving

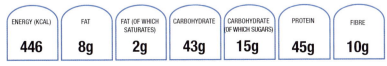

ENERGY (KCAL)	FAT	FAT (OF WHICH SATURATES)	CARBOHYDRATE	CARBOHYDRATE (OF WHICH SUGARS)	PROTEIN	FIBRE
446	8g	2g	43g	15g	45g	10g

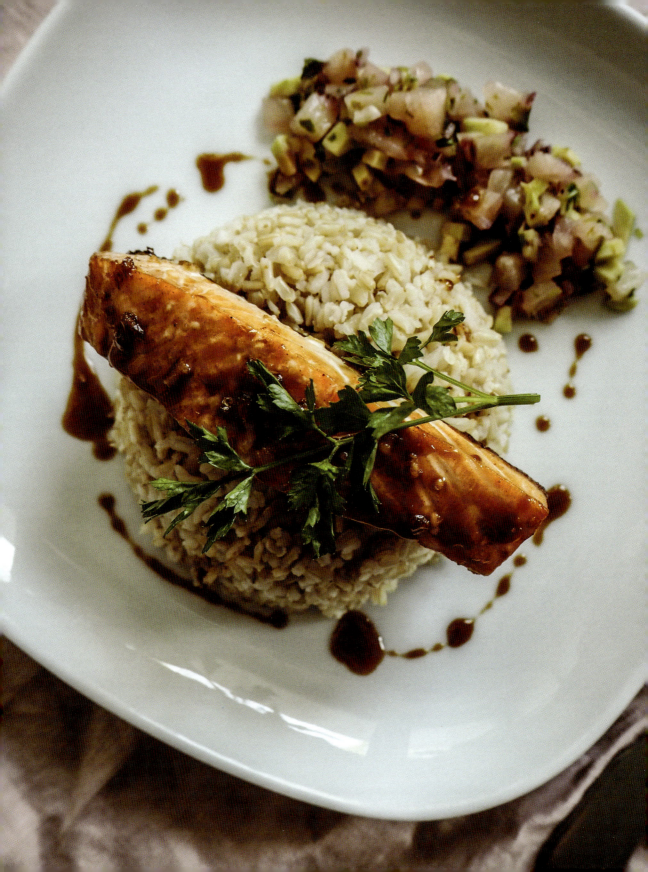

Glazed salmon

🍽 **Serves:** 4 ⏱ **Prep time:** 15 mins (plus time for marinating) 🍲 **Cooking time:** 20 mins

Ingredients

- 4 salmon fillets, skin removed

Glaze:
- Juice from 1 tin of pineapple (in natural juices, not syrup) or juice of one fresh pineapple
- 2 tbsp. reduced-salt soy sauce
- 2 garlic cloves, crushed
- Pinch of cayenne pepper

Salsa:
- ½ fresh or 1 tin pineapple cut into chunks
- 1 avocado, pitted and diced
- 1 jalapeno pepper, deseeded and diced
- ½ small red onion, diced
- 4 tbsp. fresh coriander, chopped
- Juice of half a lime

Serve with boiled brown rice, 70g/¹⁄₃ cup per person.

Method

1. In a bowl combine the ingredients for the glaze, stir together and pour over the salmon in a baking dish. Cover and chill for at least 30 minutes.

2. Combine all of the salsa ingredients and mix well. Refrigerate until ready to serve.

3. Remove the salmon from the marinade, place on a baking tray and bake in a preheated oven at 200°C/400°F (fan 180°C/350°F) or gas mark 6 for 20 minutes.

4. Cook the rice according to the packet instructions.

5. Meanwhile, place the marinade in a saucepan and boil on a medium-high heat for 5–6 minutes, until reduced by half.

6. Halfway through cooking, pour the reduced marinade over the salmon fillets and return to the oven. Cook, uncovered, until the salmon is fully cooked through.

7. Serve the salmon with salsa and boiled brown rice.

NUTRITION INFORMATION
Amount per serving

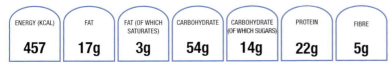

ENERGY (KCAL)	FAT	FAT (OF WHICH SATURATES)	CARBOHYDRATE	CARBOHYDRATE (OF WHICH SUGARS)	PROTEIN	FIBRE
457	17g	3g	54g	14g	22g	5g

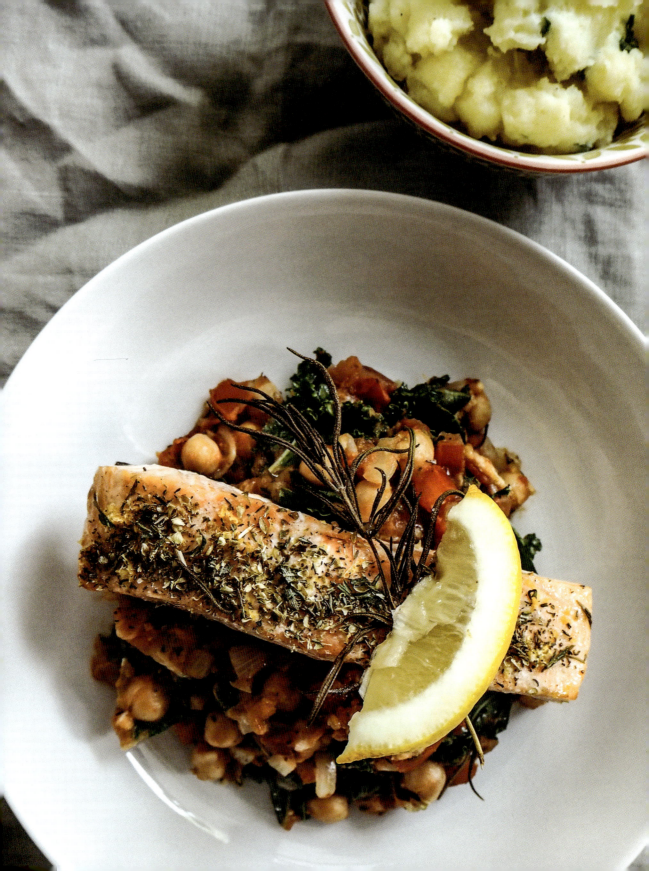

Grilled lemon-scented salmon with chickpea, tomato and spinach ragout

🍽 **Serves:** 4 ⏱ **Prep time:** 10 mins 🍲 **Cooking time:** 35 mins

Ingredients

- 1 small onion, finely diced
- 1 tsp. vegetable oil
- 2 cloves garlic, finely chopped/crushed
- 6 large plum tomatoes, roughly chopped
- 2 x 400g/14oz tins chickpeas, drained
- Fresh rosemary, parsley and thyme, chopped
- Zest and juice of 1 lemon
- Baby spinach (80g/½ cup)
- 4 salmon fillets
- Lemon cut into wedges

Serve with a portion of champ mash (see page 301) and a wedge of lemon.

Method

1. Fry the onion gently on a medium heat, without colouring, in 1 tsp. oil. Add garlic and half the chopped herbs and cook for 2–3 minutes. Add chopped tomatoes and cook on a low heat for 30 minutes.

2. Add the chickpeas, a pinch of lemon zest, a tsp. of lemon juice and the spinach and cook for a further 2–3 minutes until spinach has wilted and is combined into the ragout.

3. Place the salmon fillets on parchment paper and sprinkle over some lemon zest and the remaining chopped herbs and bake in a hot oven at 180°C/350°F (fan 160°C/320°F) or gas mark 4 for 10–15 minutes until cooked through.

4. To serve, spoon the chickpea ragout into a bowl and place the salmon fillet on top. Serve with a wedge of lemon and a portion of champ mash.

NUTRITION INFORMATION
Amount per serving

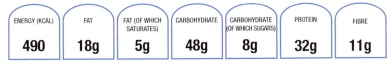

ENERGY (KCAL)	FAT	FAT (OF WHICH SATURATES)	CARBOHYDRATE	CARBOHYDRATE (OF WHICH SUGARS)	PROTEIN	FIBRE
490	18g	5g	48g	8g	32g	11g

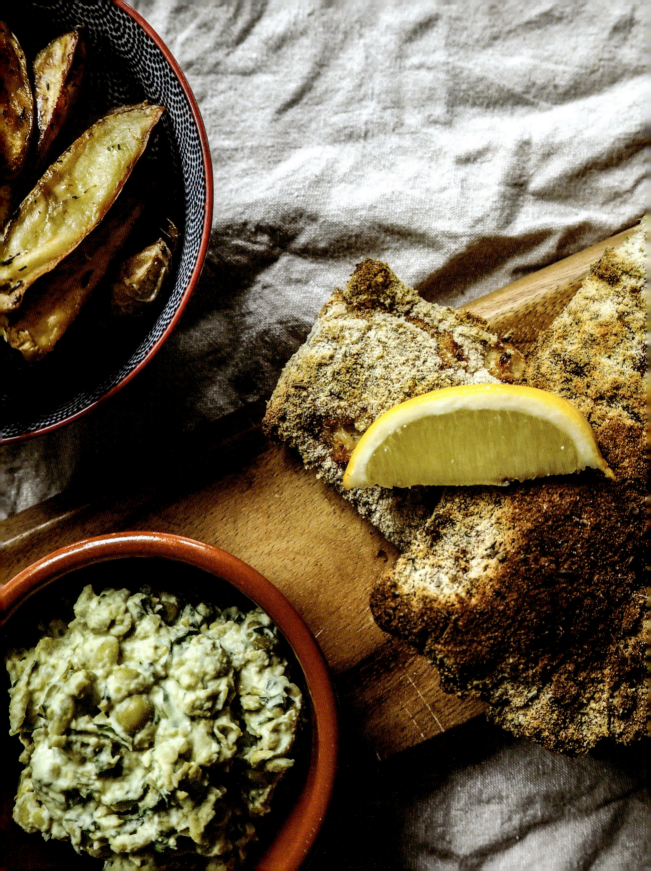

Healthy fish and chips

🍽 **Serves:** 4 ⏱ **Prep time:** 15 mins 🍲 **Cooking time:** 30 mins

Ingredients

- 120g/1¼ cups wholemeal breadcrumbs (made from wholemeal bread)
- 1 tbsp. dried herbs (mix of herbs of your choice)
- 50g/⅓ cup plain flour
- 2 eggs, whisked
- 4 raw cod fillets (500g/18oz), skin and bones removed
- 320g/2 cups frozen peas
- 1 tbsp. of fresh mint leaves
- 1 heaped tbsp. of half-fat crème fraiche
- Lemon and black pepper to season

Serve with homemade wedges (150g/5oz portion per person) (see page 307).

Method

1. Preheat the oven to 200°C/400°F (fan 180°C/350°F) or gas mark 6.

2. Place the flour, whisked eggs and breadcrumbs (mixed with the dried herbs) on three separate plates.

3. Dredge each cod fillet in the flour, then in the egg and finally in the breadcrumb and herb mix.

4. Place the fillets on a baking tray, and place in the preheated oven for 12–15 minutes until cooked through.

5. To make the mushy peas, cook the frozen peas in boiling water as per the packet instructions. Drain and mash the peas with a potato masher. Add the crème fraiche and the chopped mint, along with a squeeze of lemon and a twist of black pepper.

6. Serve the fish with the crispy wedges and minty mushy peas.

NUTRITION INFORMATION
Amount per serving

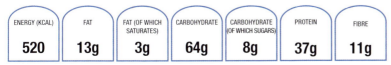

ENERGY (KCAL)	FAT	FAT (OF WHICH SATURATES)	CARBOHYDRATE	CARBOHYDRATE (OF WHICH SUGARS)	PROTEIN	FIBRE
520	13g	3g	64g	8g	37g	11g

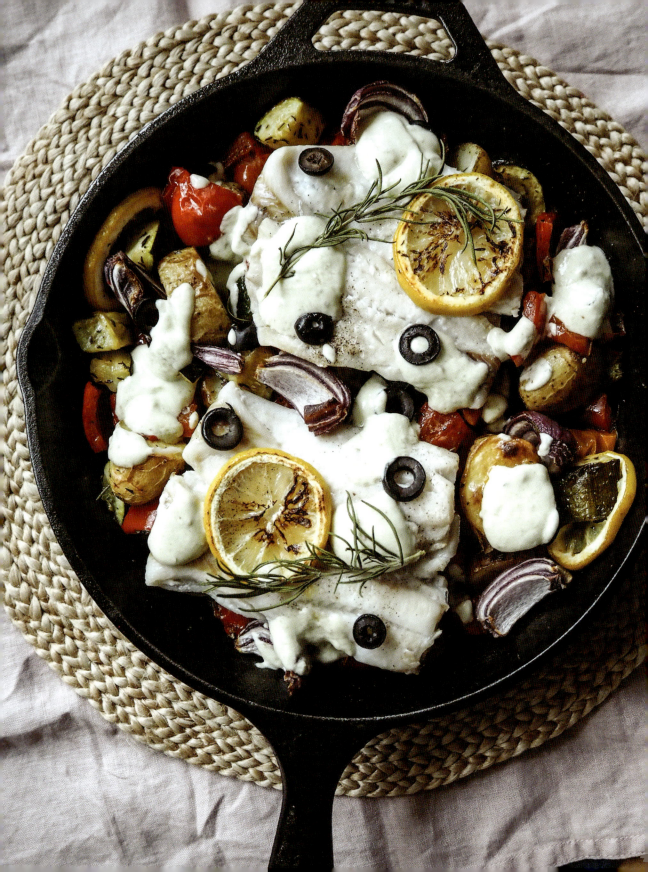

Mediterranean fish tray bake

🍽 **Serves:** 4 ⏱ **Prep time:** 15 mins 🍲 **Cooking time:** 30–35 mins

Ingredients

- 800g/28oz baby potatoes
- 250g/1¼ cups cherry tomatoes
- 1 courgette, chopped
- 2 red peppers, chopped
- 1 red onion, peeled and cut into wedges
- Handful of black olives (stones removed), rinsed
- 4 cloves of garlic, peeled and quartered
- Sprigs of fresh thyme or rosemary
- 1–2 tbsp. olive oil
- 4 x 120g/4oz fish fillets of your choice, e.g. salmon, cod, hake, etc
- ½ lemon, sliced into rounds

Dressing:
- Small handful fresh basil leaves
- Juice ½ lemon
- ½ a small clove of garlic
- ½ tsp. Dijon mustard
- 4 heaped tbsp. low-fat Greek-style yogurt
- 1 tbsp. extra virgin olive oil

Method

1. Preheat the oven to 200°C/400°F (fan 180°C/350°F) or gas mark 6.

2. Scrub the potatoes clean and halve any large ones.

3. Arrange the potatoes and all of the vegetables in a baking tray lined with grease-proof paper and scatter over the olives, herbs, garlic and 1–2 tbsp. of olive oil.

4. Place in the oven and cook for 15–20 minutes.

5. Remove the tray from the oven and place the fish fillets on top of the vegetables, along with the rounds of lemon. Return the tray to the oven and continue to cook for a further 15–20 minutes or until the potatoes, vegetables and fish are cooked through.

6. While the tray bake is cooking, make the basil and mustard yogurt dressing. Crush the basil and scrape into a bowl. Add ½ clove crushed garlic, mustard, yogurt and the juice of ½ a lemon. Add 1 tbsp. of olive oil, mix well and serve drizzled over the salmon tray bake when cooked.

NUTRITION INFORMATION
Amount per serving

ENERGY (KCAL)	FAT	FAT (OF WHICH SATURATES)	CARBOHYDRATE	CARBOHYDRATE (OF WHICH SUGARS)	PROTEIN	FIBRE
405	14g	2g	39g	12g	31g	8g

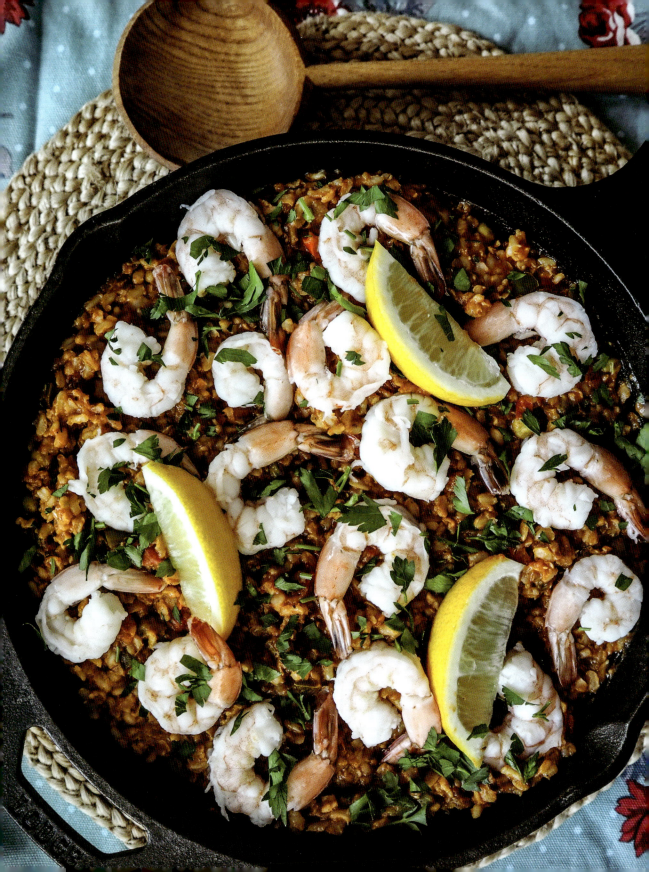

Prawn paella

🍽️ **Serves:** 4 ⏱️ **Prep time:** 15 mins 🍲 **Cooking time:** 40 mins

Ingredients

- 1 tbsp. olive oil
- 1 onion, peeled and finely chopped
- 1 red pepper, diced
- 1 green pepper, diced
- 3 cloves garlic, peeled and minced
- Pinch of saffron
- 2 tsp. hot smoked paprika
- 1 tsp. dried thyme leaves
- 1 tsp. dried oregano
- 1 tsp. cumin
- 800ml/3$\frac{1}{3}$ cups chicken stock
- 400g/14oz tin chopped tomatoes
- 300g/1½ cups brown rice
- 300g/11oz large cooked prawns
- 150g/1 cup frozen peas
- Parsley, a small bunch, chopped
- Lemon wedges to serve

Method

1. Add oil to a large saucepan over medium-high heat.

2. Add the onion, peppers and garlic. Sauté until the onions are soft.

3. Stir in the herbs and spices. Add the tinned tomatoes, stock and rice. Bring to the boil then reduce heat to low. Cover and simmer until the rice is almost tender, about 15 minutes (check recommended cooking time of the chosen rice).

4. Add the prawns and peas into the rice, then cover and cook until the prawns are fully heated through, about 6 minutes.

5. Serve garnished with parsley and a wedge of lemon.

NUTRITION INFORMATION
Amount per serving

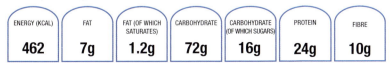

ENERGY (KCAL)	FAT	FAT (OF WHICH SATURATES)	CARBOHYDRATE	CARBOHYDRATE (OF WHICH SUGARS)	PROTEIN	FIBRE
462	7g	1.2g	72g	16g	24g	10g

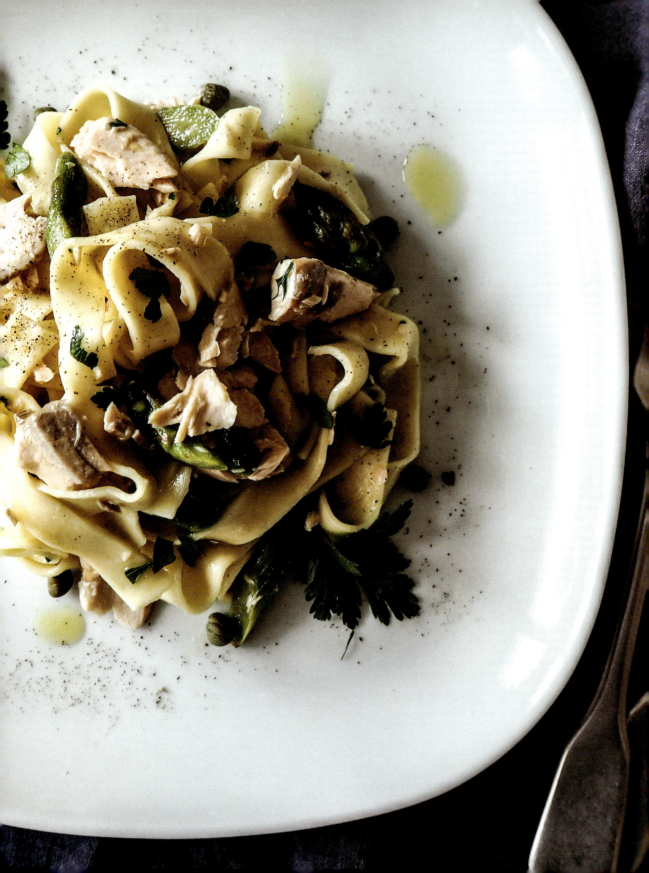

Salmon linguine

🍽 **Serves:** 2 ⏱ **Prep time:** 20 mins 🍲 **Cooking time:** 10–15 mins

Ingredients

- 225g/8oz brown spaghetti/linguine/fettuccini/tagliatelle pasta
- 250g/9oz salmon fillets
- 1 lemon, zest and juice
- 250g/2 cups asparagus
- 1 tbsp. olive oil
- 1 large clove of garlic, minced
- 150ml/¾ cup chicken stock
- 1½ tsp. capers, rinsed
- 1 tsp. cornflour mixed with 10ml/1 dessertspoon cold water
- ¼ cup chopped fresh parsley
- Freshly ground black pepper

Method

1. Cook the pasta according to the packet instructions.

2. Meanwhile cover the fish and microwave for 4 minutes or bake in the oven for 15–20 minutes at 180°C/350°F (fan 160°C/320°F) or gas mark 4. Remove skin and flake into large pieces when cooked.

3. Zest the lemon and squeeze 1–1½ tsp. juice.

4. Slice the asparagus into bite-sized pieces. Heat oil and garlic in a large saucepan over medium heat for 1 minute. Stir in the broth and capers, and allow to simmer over a low heat.

5. Stir asparagus into the simmering broth and cook for 4–7 minutes. Stir in lemon zest and juice. Mix the cornflour with water and add to the pot to thicken the broth.

6. Toss with the hot drained pasta.

7. Stir in the salmon and parsley. For extra tang, stir in more lemon. Grind black pepper over the top.

NUTRITION INFORMATION
Amount per serving

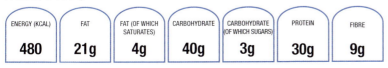

ENERGY (KCAL)	FAT	FAT (OF WHICH SATURATES)	CARBOHYDRATE	CARBOHYDRATE (OF WHICH SUGARS)	PROTEIN	FIBRE
480	21g	4g	40g	3g	30g	9g

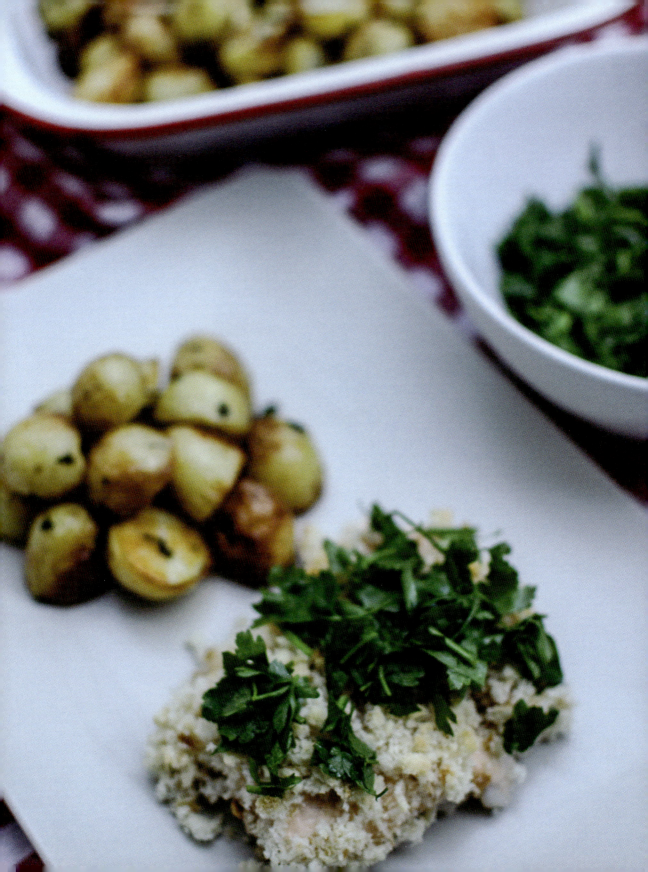

Seared haddock with horseradish aioli

🍽 **Serves:** 4 ⏱ **Prep time:** 10 mins 🍲 **Cooking time:** 15 mins

Ingredients

For the aioli:
- 5 tbsp. low-fat mayonnaise
- 2 tsp. horseradish sauce
- ¾ tsp. lemon juice
- 1 garlic clove, minced
- ½ tsp. tomato puree
- Black pepper

For the fish:
- 3 tbsp. rapeseed oil
- 4 skinless haddock fillets, about 120g/4oz each
- Black pepper
- 100g/1 cup dry wholemeal breadcrumbs
- 2 handfuls of fresh parsley, chopped
- Juice of ½ lemon
- Serve with roast garlic baby potatoes (see page 305)
- Mixed salad

Method

1. Preheat the oven to 220°C/425°F (fan 200°C/400°F) or gas mark 7. Mix the aioli ingredients in a small bowl and season with black pepper. Cover and refrigerate.

2. Heat 1 tbsp. oil in a large, non-stick frying pan over a medium-high heat. Pat the fish fillets dry with kitchen paper and season with black pepper. When the pan is hot, cook the fillets for two minutes; be careful not to move them.

3. When they are nicely browned, flip the fillets over and remove the pan from the heat. Transfer the fish to an ovenproof baking dish.

4. Spread the seared side of each fillet with some aioli mixture and then top with a layer of breadcrumbs.

5. Place the tray in the oven and bake for 10–15 minutes, or until the fish is cooked through.

6. Meanwhile, combine the parsley leaves, lemon juice and 2 tbsp. of oil in a bowl.

7. When the fish is cooked, remove the tray from the oven and transfer the fillets to plates. Top each with some of the parsley salad and serve warm with roast garlic baby potatoes.

NUTRITION INFORMATION
Amount per serving

ENERGY (KCAL)	FAT	FAT (OF WHICH SATURATES)	CARBOHYDRATE	CARBOHYDRATE (OF WHICH SUGARS)	PROTEIN	FIBRE
507	15g	2g	62g	7g	30g	7g

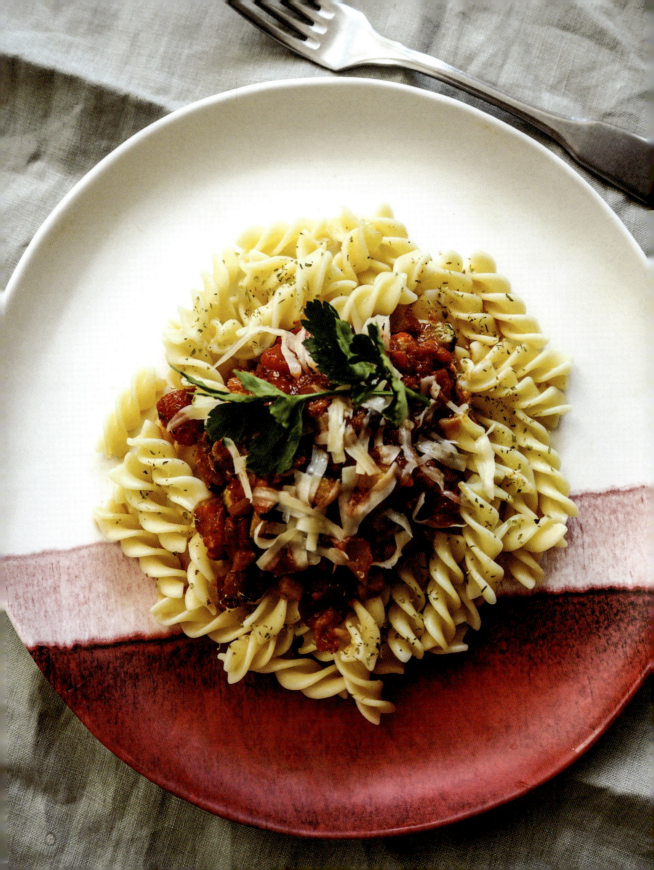

Pasta with mackerel and Mediterranean vegetables

🍽 **Serves:** 4 ⏱ **Prep time:** 10 mins 🍲 **Cooking time:** 15 mins

Ingredients

- 1 tbsp. rapeseed oil
- 2 cloves garlic, crushed
- 1 large onion, peeled and chopped
- 6 mushrooms, washed and sliced
- 1 red pepper, chopped
- 1 courgette, diced
- 2 small tins mackerel in tomato sauce (250g/9oz)
- 1 tin chopped tomatoes (400g/14oz)
- 1 tbsp. tomato puree (15g/½oz)
- Pinch of sugar
- 1 tsp. dried oregano
- 400g/4 cups wholewheat pasta

Method

1. Cook the pasta according to the packet instructions.

2. Heat the oil in a large pan or wok. Add the garlic and vegetables and sauté until soft.

3. Add the tinned mackerel, tomatoes, tomato puree, sugar and oregano, and simmer for 10 minutes. Add a little water if the sauce is too thick.

4. Add the pasta to the sauce, mix well and serve in warm bowls.

NUTRITION INFORMATION
Amount per serving

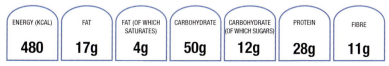

ENERGY (KCAL)	FAT	FAT (OF WHICH SATURATES)	CARBOHYDRATE	CARBOHYDRATE (OF WHICH SUGARS)	PROTEIN	FIBRE
480	17g	4g	50g	12g	28g	11g

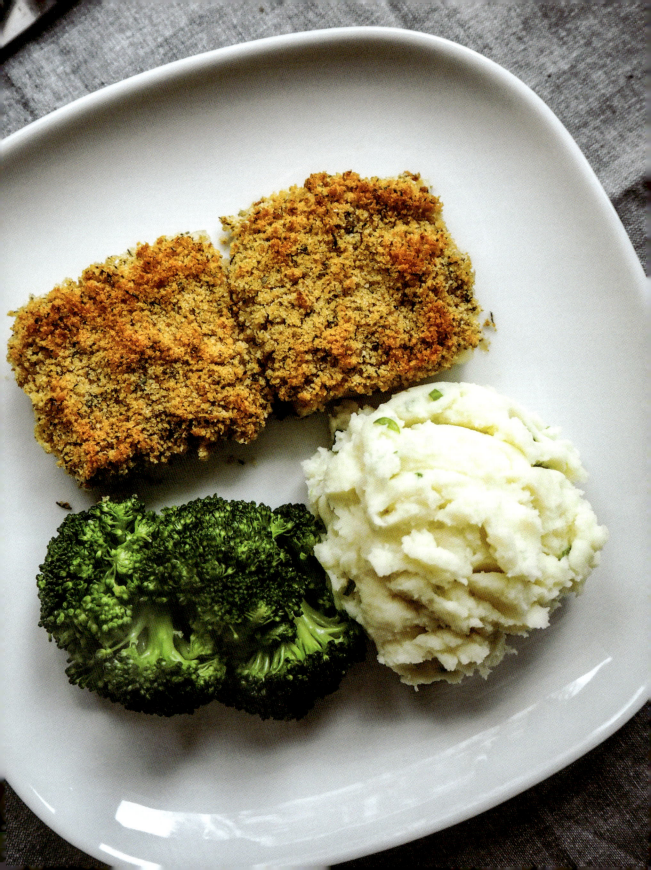

Baked hake/cod with a herb crust

🍽 **Serves:** 2 ⏱ **Prep time:** 5 mins 🍲 **Cooking time:** 15–20 mins

Ingredients

- 2 fillets of cod or hake (240g/9oz)
- 50g/½ cup breadcrumbs
- 2 tsp. olive oil
- 1 tsp. herbs (parsley and chives)
- Freshly ground black pepper
- Squeeze of lemon

Serve with a portion of champ mash (see page 301) and green vegetables of choice.

Method

1. Place the fish on a baking tray lined with baking parchment.

2. Mix the breadcrumbs, finely chopped herbs and oil. Press the breadcrumbs onto the fish fillets.

3. Bake at 180°C/350°F (fan 160°C/320°F) or gas mark 4 for 12–15 minutes.

4. Season with freshly ground black pepper and a squeeze of lemon and serve with champ mash and green vegetables of choice.

NUTRITION INFORMATION
Amount per serving

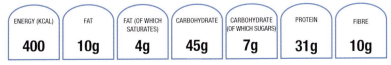

ENERGY (KCAL)	FAT	FAT (OF WHICH SATURATES)	CARBOHYDRATE	CARBOHYDRATE (OF WHICH SUGARS)	PROTEIN	FIBRE
400	10g	4g	45g	7g	31g	10g

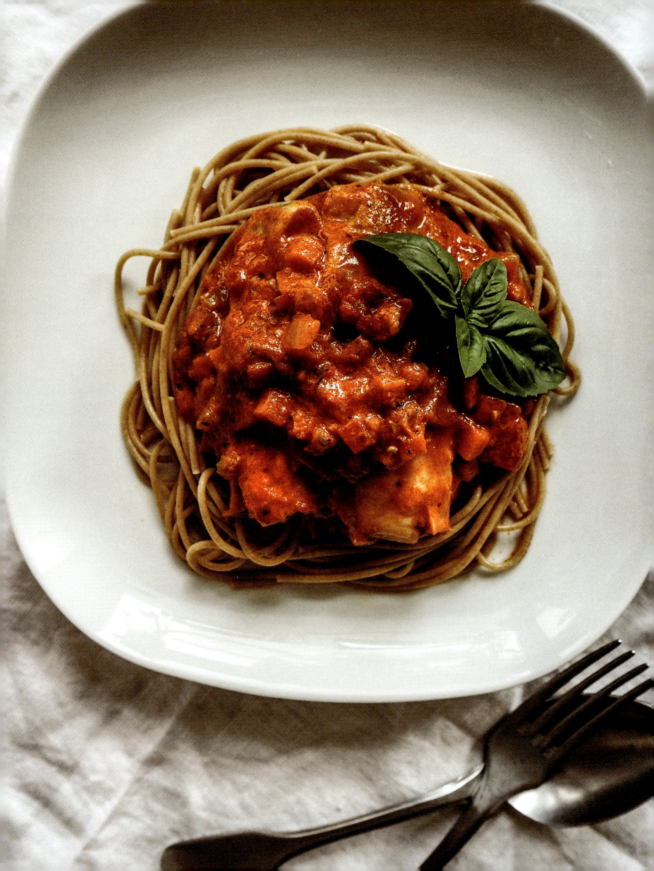

Spicy Italian cod

Serves: 4 **Prep time:** 15 mins **Cooking time:** 30 mins

Ingredients

- Wholewheat spaghetti (80–100g/3–3 ½oz raw per person)
- 2 small carrots, roughly chopped
- 2 stalks of celery, roughly chopped
- 1 small onion, roughly chopped
- 2 tsp. olive oil
- 1 tbsp. tomato puree
- 1 tsp. paprika
- 1 tsp. ground chilli powder
- 1 tsp. dried oregano
- 2 cloves garlic, peeled and finely chopped
- 2 x 400g/14oz tins chopped tomatoes
- 1 tsp. pepper
- 4 x 160g/6oz cod fillets
- 2 tbsp. low-fat crème fraiche (30ml/1oz)
- Small handful fresh basil leaves

Method

1. Cook the spaghetti according to the packet instructions and drain well.

2. Place the carrots, celery and onion in a food processor and blend until they are finely chopped.

3. Heat the olive oil in a large pan. Add the carrot, celery and onion and cook over a medium heat for 2 minutes to soften.

4. Add the tomato puree with the paprika, chilli powder, dried oregano and garlic. Cook for another 3 minutes, stirring gently. Stir in the tinned tomatoes and bring to the boil for 5 minutes, then turn down to a gentle simmer. Add pepper to season.

5. Add the fish fillets, ensuring they are covered by the sauce. Leave the mixture to simmer over a low heat for 10–15 minutes until the fish is cooked. Finish the sauce with the crème fraiche.

6. Place a large spoonful of spaghetti onto the middle of the plate to serve. Spoon over the sauce and one fish fillet per person. Garnish with basil.

NUTRITION INFORMATION
Amount per serving

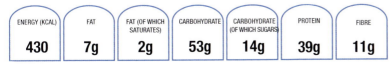

ENERGY (KCAL)	FAT	FAT (OF WHICH SATURATES)	CARBOHYDRATE	CARBOHYDRATE (OF WHICH SUGARS)	PROTEIN	FIBRE
430	7g	2g	53g	14g	39g	11g

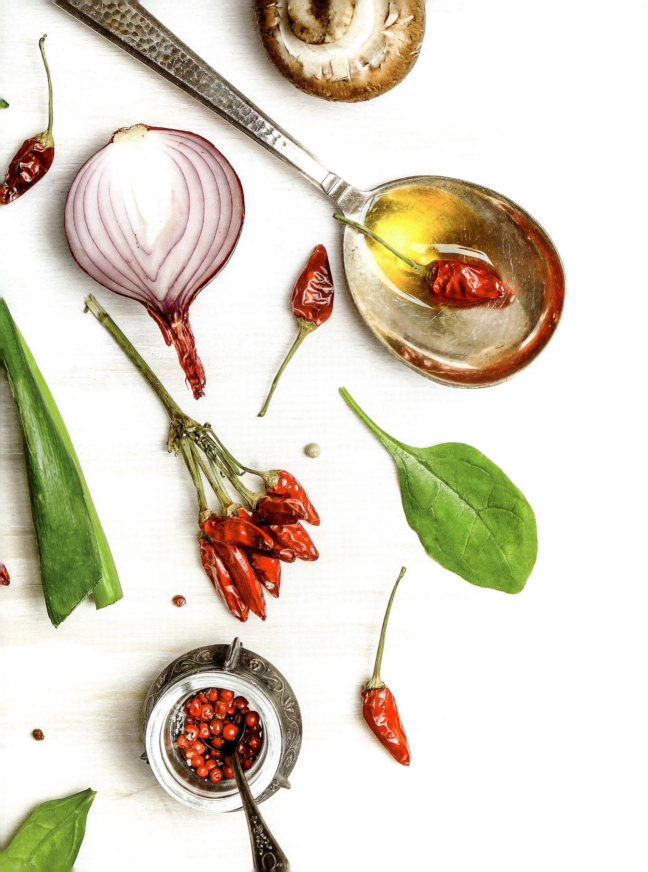

Vegetarian

Bean chilli

Butternut squash, chickpea and spinach curry

Pasta arrabbiata

Egg-fried rice

Healthy pizza

Millet, sweet potato and cashew burgers

Kidney bean and potato curry

Ratatouille

Roast tomato and orzo bake

Stuffed mushrooms

Vegetable and red lentil pie

Vegetable jalfrezi

Butter bean stew

Kale, tomato and lemon spaghetti

Vegetarian casserole

Quorn pie

Spicy rice and lentil one-pot

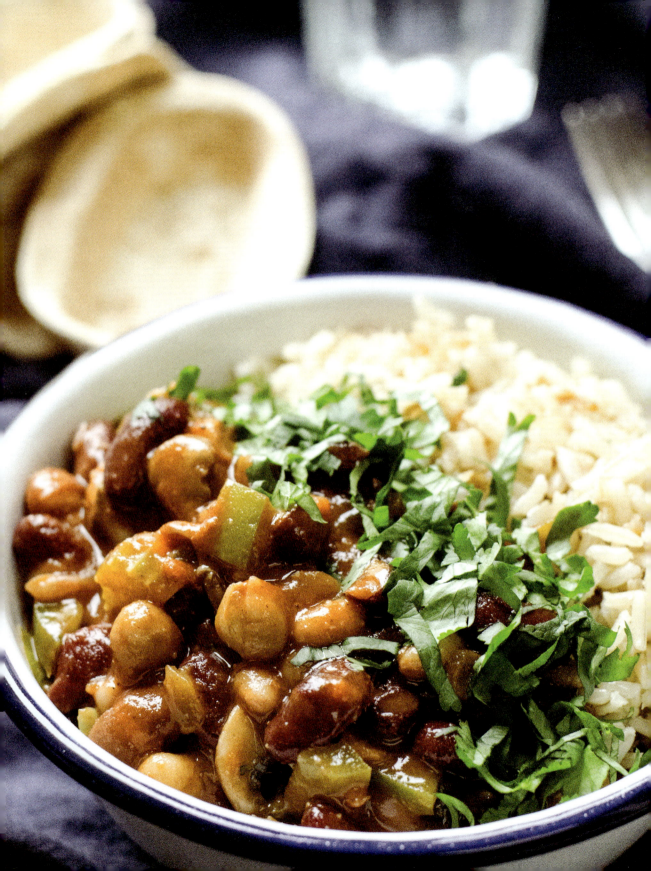

Bean chilli

🍽 **Serves:** 8 ⏱ **Prep time:** 20–25 mins ♨ **Cooking time:** 30–40 mins

Ingredients

- 1 tbsp. olive or rapeseed oil
- 2 onions, peeled and chopped
- 4 cloves garlic, peeled and crushed
- 1 large red pepper, diced
- 1 large green pepper, diced
- 200g/2½ cups mushrooms, washed and sliced
- 2 small carrots, diced
- 2 sticks celery, diced
- 1 tsp. chilli powder (reduce or increase to taste) or use finely chopped fresh chilli
- 1 tsp. cumin
- 1 tsp. ground coriander
- 2 x 400g/14oz tins chopped tomatoes
- 1 tin kidney beans, drained
- 1 tin baked beans in tomato sauce
- 100g/²⁄₃ cup frozen sweetcorn
- 1 tin chickpeas, drained
- 4 tbsp. tomato puree
- Chopped coriander to serve

Serve with a portion of brown rice
(70g/¹⁄₃ cup per person) or a baked potato.

Method

1. Heat the oil in a large pan or wok. Add all the prepared vegetables and spices and sauté for 10 minutes until the vegetables are soft.

2. Add the remaining ingredients, stir to mix well. Cover and leave to simmer for 20 minutes.

3. Sprinkle with chopped coriander and serve with brown rice.

4. Note: This dish freezes well. You can vary the beans used depending on what you have in your cupboard, e.g. cannellini beans/butter beans.

NUTRITION INFORMATION
Amount per serving

ENERGY (KCAL)	FAT	FAT (OF WHICH SATURATES)	CARBOHYDRATE	CARBOHYDRATE (OF WHICH SUGARS)	PROTEIN	FIBRE
375	5g	1g	66g	13g	15g	13g

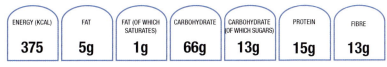

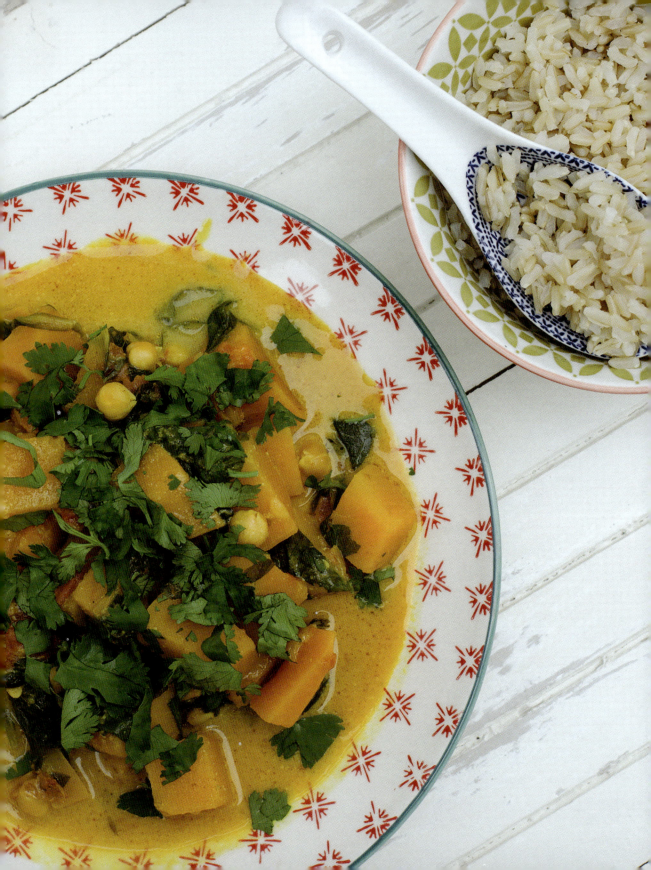

Butternut squash, chickpea and spinach curry

🍽 **Serves:** 6 ⏱ **Prep time:** 20 mins 🍲 **Cooking time:** 30 mins

Ingredients

- 1 butternut squash
- 200g/1 cup spinach leaves
- 20ml/2 dessertspoons sunflower oil
- 1 tsp. cumin seeds
- 1 tsp. brown mustard seeds
- 1 onion, chopped
- 2 large cloves garlic, chopped finely
- 1 green chilli, deseeded and chopped finely
- 2½cm/1in fresh ginger, peeled and chopped
- 1 heaped tsp. turmeric
- 2 tsp. ground coriander
- 1 x 400g/14oz tin of chopped tomatoes
- 1 x 400g/14oz tin of chickpeas, rinsed and drained
- 400ml/14oz tin of light coconut milk
- 200ml/1 cup water
- Handful of fresh coriander, roughly chopped
- Lemon juice, to taste
- Brown rice, cooked as per packet instructions (75g/¹⁄₃ cup uncooked per person)

Method

1. Peel the butternut squash, remove the seeds and chop into 1in pieces.

2. Remove and discard any thick stalks from the spinach. Wash and roughly chop the leaves.

3. Heat the oil over a medium heat. Add the cumin seeds and mustard seeds and allow to pop for 2 minutes.

4. Add the onion and fry until soft, about 5 minutes. Add the garlic, chilli, ginger, ground coriander and turmeric, and stir for a further minute. Add the butternut squash, tomatoes and 200ml/1 cup water.

5. Bring to a boil, lower the heat, cover and cook for 15 minutes.

6. Add the coconut milk, chickpeas and spinach leaves. Cover and cook for a further 5 minutes or until the squash and spinach are tender.

7. Stir in the fresh coriander and season with a little lemon juice to taste. Serve with a portion of brown rice.

NUTRITION INFORMATION
Amount per serving

ENERGY (KCAL)	FAT	FAT (OF WHICH SATURATES)	CARBOHYDRATE	CARBOHYDRATE (OF WHICH SUGARS)	PROTEIN	FIBRE
420	11g	5g	63g	9g	15g	12g

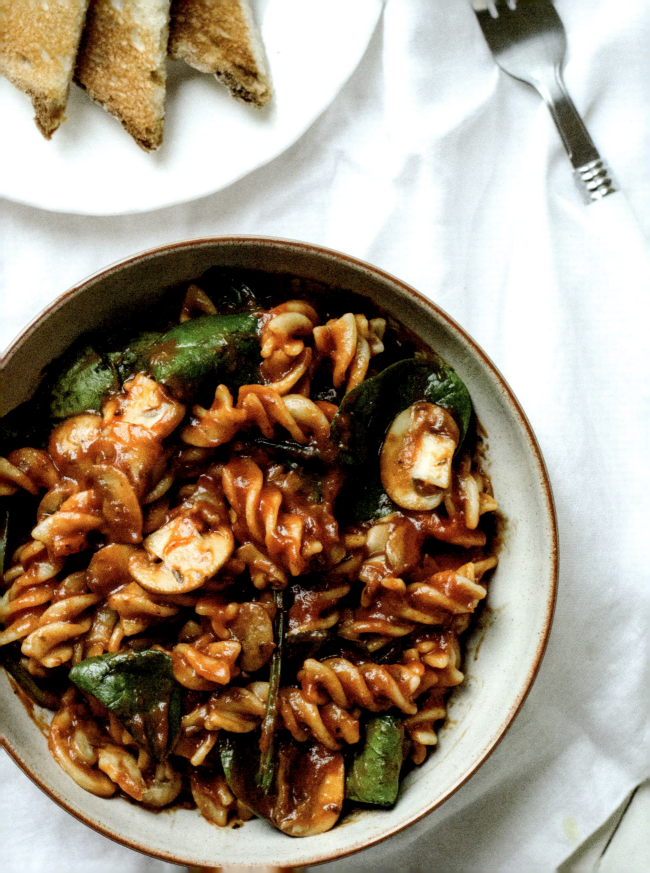

Pasta arrabbiata

Serves: 4 **Prep time:** 10 mins **Cooking time:** 15 mins

Ingredients

- 400g/4 cups brown pasta
- 2 heaped tsp. dried oregano
- 2 heaped tsp. dried thyme
- 2 heaped tsp. chilli flakes
- 4 garlic cloves, crushed
- 2 tbsp. olive oil
- 24 cherry tomatoes (~350g/1¾ cups), cut into quarters
- 2 x 400g/14oz tin chopped tomatoes
- 400g/5⅓ cups mushrooms, washed and sliced
- 2 tbsp. tomato puree
- 100g/½ cup spinach
- Juice 1 lemon

Method

1. Cook the pasta as per the packet instructions.

2. Heat the dried oregano, thyme, chilli and garlic in a frying pan with the oil.

3. Add the mushrooms, tomatoes, tinned tomatoes and tomato puree. Cook for 5–7 minutes, until the cherry tomatoes are soft.

4. Stir in the spinach and allow to wilt.

5. Add the lemon juice and season with pepper.

6. When the pasta is cooked, stir it into the sauce.

NUTRITION INFORMATION
Amount per serving

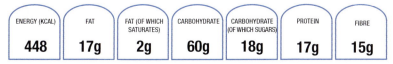

ENERGY (KCAL)	FAT	FAT (OF WHICH SATURATES)	CARBOHYDRATE	CARBOHYDRATE (OF WHICH SUGARS)	PROTEIN	FIBRE
448	17g	2g	60g	18g	17g	15g

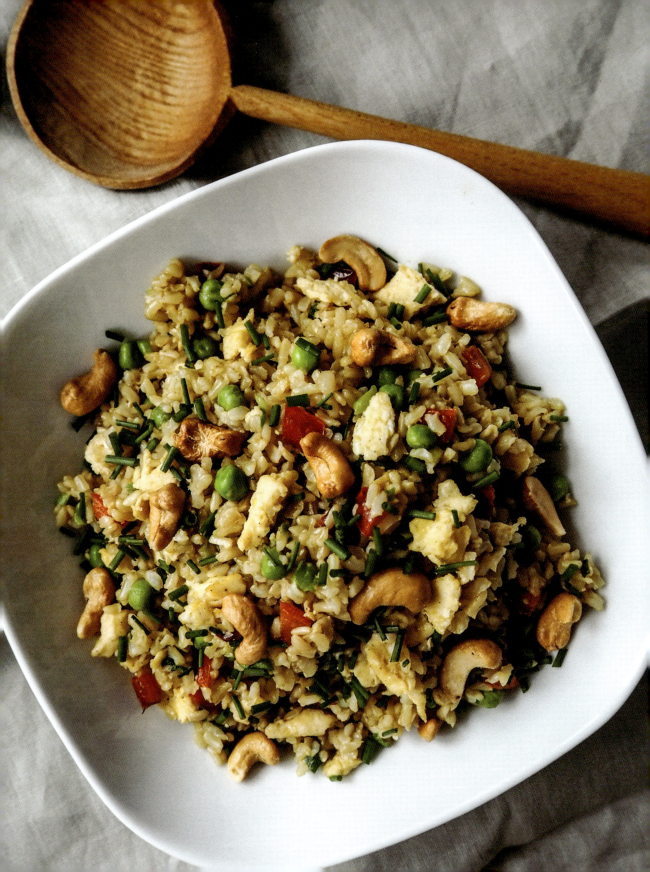

Egg-fried rice

🍽 **Serves:** 4 ⏱ **Prep time:** 10 mins 🍲 **Cooking time:** 8 mins

Ingredients

- 200g/1 cup brown rice
- 150g/1 cup frozen peas
- 2 large eggs
- Freshly ground black pepper
- 2 tbsp. sunflower oil
- 1 red pepper, deseeded and diced
- 8 spring onions, trimmed and thinly sliced
- 2 garlic cloves, finely chopped
- 2 tsp. five-spice powder
- 3 tbsp. reduced-sodium soy sauce mixed with 2 tbsp. water
- 140g/1½ cups bean sprouts
- 1 tbsp. snipped fresh chives
- 50g/⅓ cup roasted cashew nuts (unsalted)

Method

1. Cook the brown rice and frozen peas as per packet instructions.

2. While they are cooking, beat the eggs and season with freshly ground black pepper.

3. Heat 1 tbsp. of oil in a frying pan over medium-high heat until hot. Add the eggs and cook for 2 minutes. Remove the omelette to a chopping board and thinly slice.

4. Add the remaining oil, pepper, onion, garlic and spices to the wok. Stir-fry for 3–4 minutes.

5. Reduce the heat and stir in the soy sauce mix, bean sprouts, sliced omelette, cooked rice and peas. Gently stir-fry for 1–2 minutes or until heated through. Finally, stir in the chives and cashew nuts and serve.

NUTRITION INFORMATION
Amount per serving

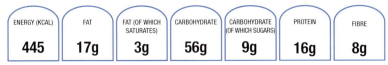

ENERGY (KCAL)	FAT	FAT (OF WHICH SATURATES)	CARBOHYDRATE	CARBOHYDRATE (OF WHICH SUGARS)	PROTEIN	FIBRE
445	17g	3g	56g	9g	16g	8g

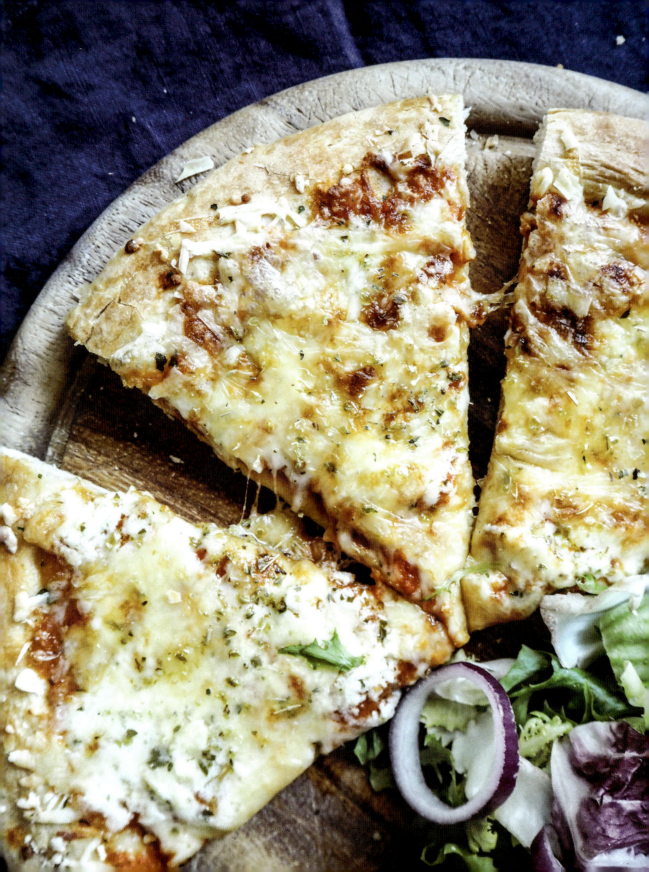

Healthy pizza

Serves: Makes 3 pizzas

Prep time: 15 mins **Cooking time:** 20 mins plus 1 hour proving time for dough

Ingredients

**Pizza base
(makes 3 pizza bases):**
- 500g/4 cups strong flour
- Pinch of salt
- 1 tbsp. olive oil
- 15g/½oz fresh yeast or 5g/2 tsp. dried yeast
- 300ml/1¼ cups warm water
- 5g/1 tsp. caster sugar

Tomato sauce:
- 1 tbsp. olive oil
- 1 tsp. tomato puree
- Pinch sugar
- 2 cloves garlic, crushed
- 2 x 400g/14oz tins tomatoes
- Freshly ground black pepper

Toppings:
- Any selection of toppings of your choice can be used on the pizza
- Vegetables: such as onions, peppers, mushrooms, finely sliced
- Meat: shredded chicken/turkey
- Cheese: mozzarella cheese; cheddar/parmesan cheese can also be used. Choose low-fat varieties.

Analysis based on toppings:
sweetcorn, peppers, mushrooms, rocket, cheese (60g/½cup).
One portion = half a pizza with a large mixed salad.

Method

1. Sieve the flour and salt into a bowl.

2. Dissolve the yeast in the water, then add the olive oil and sugar.

3. Mix the yeast mixture into the flour to form a smooth dough, place into a clean bowl and cover.

4. When doubled in size, divide the dough into 3 pieces, roll each piece out into a thin disc and place on a lightly greased baking sheet.

5. To make the tomato sauce, heat the oil in a pan and cook the garlic gently until soft but not coloured.

6. Add the tomatoes, tomato puree, sugar and seasoning and simmer for about 30 minutes until thickened.

7. Arrange the sauce and selected toppings on top and bake at 200°C/400°F (fan 180°C/350°F) or gas mark 6 for about 10 minutes.

NUTRITION INFORMATION
Amount per serving

ENERGY (KCAL)	FAT	FAT (OF WHICH SATURATES)	CARBOHYDRATE	CARBOHYDRATE (OF WHICH SUGARS)	PROTEIN	FIBRE
488	9.7g	3.8g	75g	12g	22g	6.2g

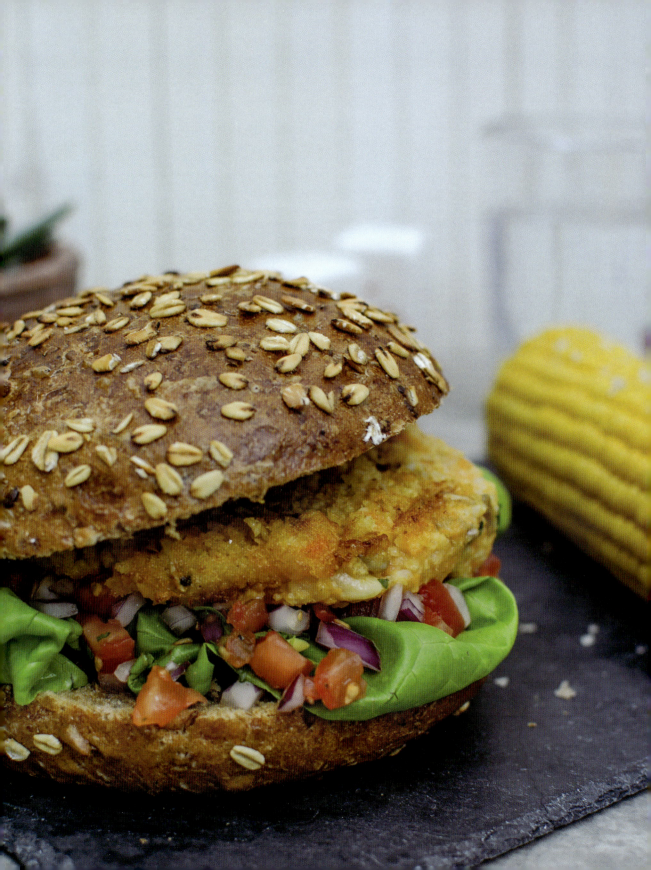

Millet, sweet potato and cashew burgers

Serves: 6 **Prep time:** 40 mins (plus 2 hours for burgers to chill in fridge)
Cooking time: 20 mins

Ingredients

For the burgers:
- 150g/¾ cup millet
- 150g/5oz sweet potato
- 150g/5oz cauliflower
- 25g/1oz cashew nuts, toasted
- 25g/½ cup carrot, roughly grated
- 25g/¼ cup sunflower seeds, toasted
- ½ tsp. ginger, finely grated
- ½ tsp. ground cumin
- 1 tsp. fresh parsley, chopped
- 2 tsp. soy sauce
- Unrefined sunflower oil, for frying
- Wholemeal bun

For the salsa:
- 4 tomatoes
- 1 small red onion, finely chopped
- 1 small red chilli, deseeded and finely chopped
- 2 tsp. fresh coriander, finely chopped
- Pepper
- Squeeze lemon juice

For the pesto (makes a batch for storing):
- 30g/¼ cup sunflower seeds, toasted
- 55g/2oz basil leaves or coriander leaves
- 1 clove garlic, chopped
- 125ml/½ cup unrefined sunflower oil
- 250ml/1 cup extra virgin olive oil

Method

1. Wash the millet well, drain and place in a heavy-bottomed pot. Peel and chop the sweet potato into 1cm/½in cubes. Divide the cauliflower into florets.

2. Add both to the millet in the pot with 300ml/1¼ cups of water. Cover and bring to a boil. Lower the heat (use a flame cover if you have one), and simmer for 30 minutes.

3. To make the salsa, cut a small x into the top of each tomato and place in a bowl of boiling water for 2 minutes. Rinse under cold water. The skins should slide off. Chop the tomatoes into small dice. Place in a bowl with the red onion, chilli, fresh coriander. Season with pepper and fresh lemon juice. Mix well.

4. To make the pesto, place the sunflower seeds into a food processor with the basil or coriander leaves and the garlic. Mix the oils together and, with the motor running, pour the oil slowly into the feeder tube of the food processor and blend.

5. Once cooked, stir the millet and vegetables well.

6. Transfer into a large bowl. Roughly chop the cashew nuts. Add to the millet along with the grated carrot, sunflower seeds, grated ginger, cumin powder, parsley and soy sauce. Mix well.

7. Divide the mix into 6 portions. Dampen your hands with water and shape the portions into burgers. Place in the fridge to set for about 2 hours.

8. Heat 2 tbsp. of sunflower oil in a pan. Fry the burgers on both sides until golden brown.

9. Serve on a wholemeal bun with 3–4 tbsp. salsa, 1 tsp. pesto and a large side salad.

NUTRITION INFORMATION
Amount per serving

ENERGY (KCAL)	FAT	FAT (OF WHICH SATURATES)	CARBOHYDRATE	CARBOHYDRATE (OF WHICH SUGARS)	PROTEIN	FIBRE
430	19g	3g	51g	12g	12g	6g

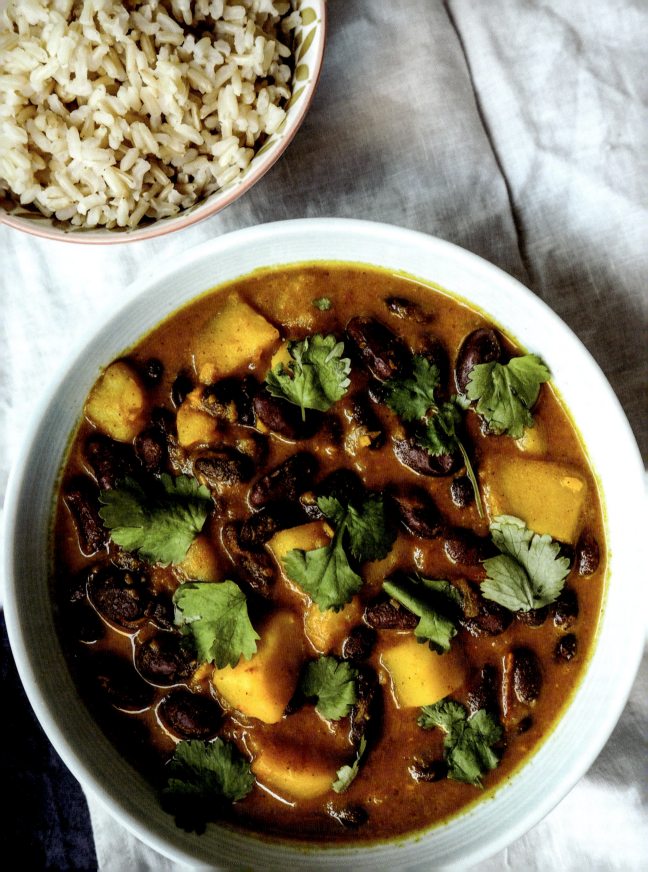

Kidney bean and potato curry

🍽 **Serves:** 4 ⏱ **Prep time:** 20 mins 🍲 **Cooking time:** 45 mins–1 hour

Ingredients

- 3 cloves of garlic, peeled
- 2cm/¾in cube fresh ginger, peeled
- 1 medium onion, finely chopped
- 1 medium tomato, finely chopped
- 4 tbsp. olive oil or rapeseed oil
- 3 large potatoes
- 1 tsp. ground turmeric
- 1½ tbsp. medium curry powder
- 2 x 400g/14oz tins kidney beans (or bean of choice), drained and rinsed
- 300ml/1¼ cups stock
- A small bunch of coriander
- Freshly ground black pepper
- 280g/1¼ cups brown rice

Method

1. Crush the garlic and ginger together in a pestle and mortar.

2. Put the oil into a wide-bottomed pan and heat over a high heat for 3 minutes.

3. When the oil is hot, turn down the heat and add the onions and tomatoes. Simmer for 5 minutes with the lid on, stirring occasionally. Add the garlic and ginger and continue to simmer for a further 5–7 minutes with the lid on, stirring occasionally.

4. Meanwhile, cut the potatoes into medium wedges and put the kettle on to boil.

5. Add the turmeric and curry powder to the pan of onions and tomatoes and stir well. Simmer for 3 minutes, still on a low to medium heat and stirring frequently. Add a tbsp. of water if anything starts to stick.

6. Add the beans, potatoes and hot stock, and stir well so that the potatoes and beans are coated in the sauce. Turn the heat up, bring to the boil, then reduce to simmer for 30–40 minutes.

7. Stir every 10 minutes to ensure the potatoes cook evenly.

8. Cook brown rice according to the packet instructions.

9. Finely chop the coriander and add to the pan a few minutes before serving and season to taste.

NUTRITION INFORMATION
Amount per serving

ENERGY (KCAL)	FAT	FAT (OF WHICH SATURATES)	CARBOHYDRATE	CARBOHYDRATE (OF WHICH SUGARS)	PROTEIN	FIBRE
535	15g	1g	80g	6g	17g	17g

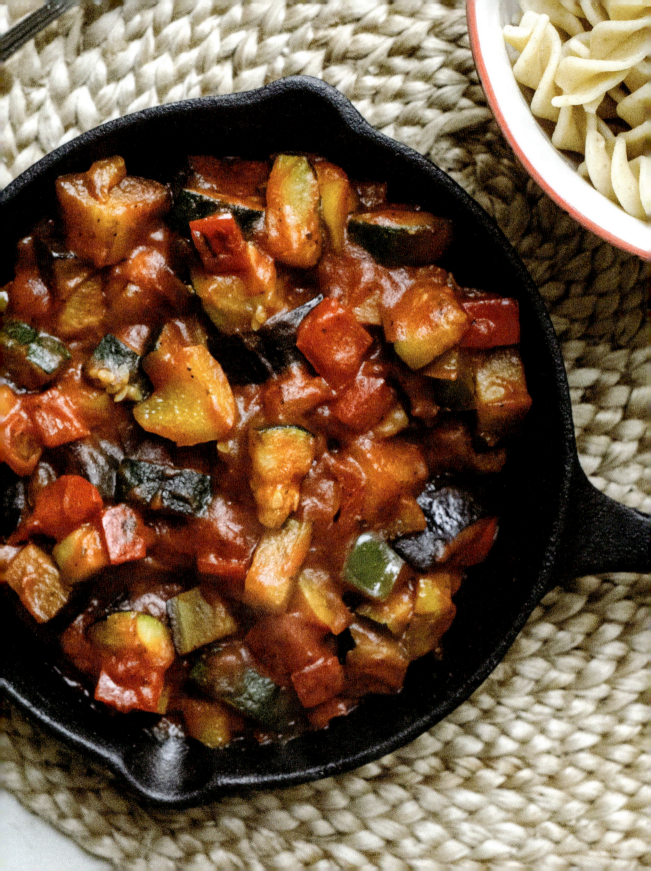

Ratatouille

|O| **Serves:** 4 ⏱ **Prep time:** 15 mins ♨ **Cooking time:** 25 mins

Ingredients

- 1 courgette, chopped
- 1 red and 1 yellow pepper, chopped
- 1 red onion, chopped
- 1 aubergine, chopped
- 2 tbsp. olive oil
- Pepper

Serve with a portion of tomato sauce (see page 187) and a portion of brown pasta (150g/¾ cup cooked).

Method

1. Toss all the vegetables in the olive oil. Season and place on a tray.

2. Bake at 200°C/400°F (fan 180°C/350°F) or gas mark 6 for 25 minutes.

3. Mix the cooked vegetables with some tomato sauce (see page 187) and a portion of cooked brown pasta.

NUTRITION INFORMATION
Amount per serving

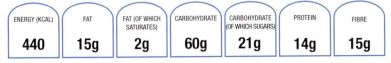

ENERGY (KCAL)	FAT	FAT (OF WHICH SATURATES)	CARBOHYDRATE	CARBOHYDRATE (OF WHICH SUGARS)	PROTEIN	FIBRE
440	15g	2g	60g	21g	14g	15g

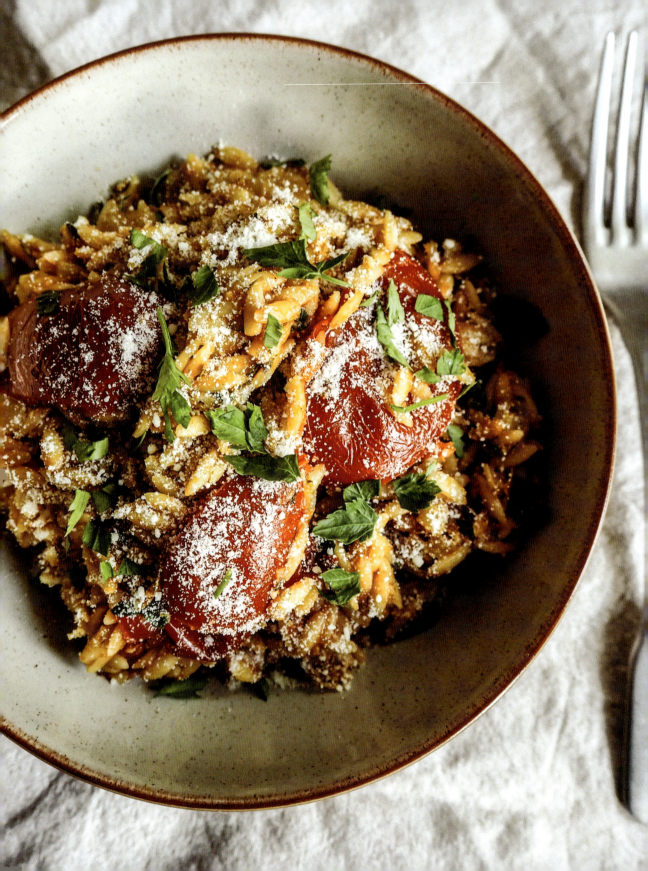

Roast tomato and orzo bake

🍽 **Serves:** 4 ⏱ **Prep time:** 15 mins 🍲 **Cooking time:** 40 mins

Ingredients

- 350g/1¾ cups ripe tomatoes, chopped into quarters
- 1 tbsp. olive oil
- Freshly ground black pepper
- 1 onion, chopped
- 1 clove garlic, chopped
- 150g/5oz courgette, ends trimmed off and grated
- 2 celery stalks, trimmed and diced
- 1–2 tsp. fennel seeds
- 1 sprig of rosemary, finely chopped
- 1 tbsp. tomato puree
- 300g/1⅔ cups orzo pasta
- 600ml/2½ cups vegetable stock
- ½ bunch fresh parsley, roughly chopped
- 30g/⅓ cup parmesan, grated

Method

1. Preheat the oven to 190°C/375°F (fan 170°C /325°F) or gas mark 5.

2. Place the tomatoes on a baking tray, drizzle over half the oil and season with pepper. Roast in the preheated oven for 20 minutes or until the tomatoes begin to collapse and colour a little.

3. Meanwhile, heat the remaining oil in a large, ovenproof casserole dish over a medium to high heat. When hot, add the onion, garlic, courgette and celery. Keep stirring the vegetables and cook for approximately 10 minutes until they have softened.

4. Add the fennel seeds, rosemary and tomato puree.

5. Remove the roasted tomatoes from the oven but don't turn off the heat. Slide the tomatoes and their juices straight from the tray into the casserole.

6. Stir in the orzo and add the stock. Bring the pot up to a simmer.

7. Cover with a lid and bake in the preheated oven for 20 minutes or until all the liquid has been absorbed and the orzo is cooked through.

8. Let the pasta sit for 5 minutes and then stir through the parsley and parmesan before serving.

NUTRITION INFORMATION
Amount per serving

ENERGY (KCAL)	FAT	FAT (OF WHICH SATURATES)	CARBOHYDRATE	CARBOHYDRATE (OF WHICH SUGARS)	PROTEIN	FIBRE
400	8g	3g	62g	7g	18g	5g

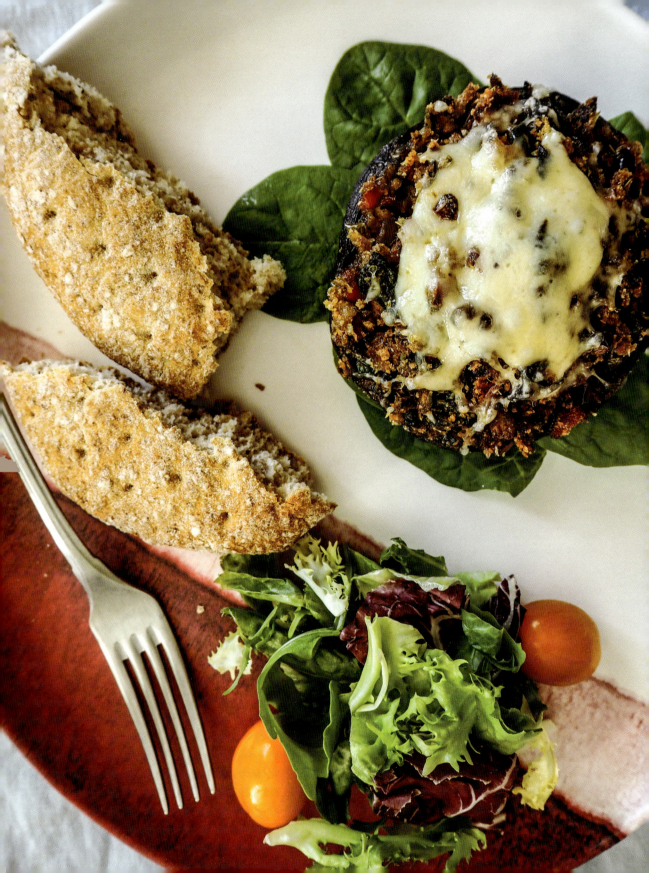

Stuffed mushrooms

🍽 **Serves:** 4 ⏱ **Prep time:** 15 mins 🍲 **Cooking time:** 10 + 20 mins

Ingredients

- 6–8 large portobello mushrooms, wiped with a damp paper towel and stalks trimmed
- 2 tbsp. olive oil
- 1 onion, diced
- 2 medium courgettes, diced
- 1 red pepper, diced
- 4 sun-dried tomatoes, drained and chopped
- 2–3 cloves garlic, minced
- Large handful of spinach
- Pinch of dried oregano, crushed between your fingers
- Dash of crushed chilli flakes
- Freshly ground black pepper, to taste
- 100g/1 cup wholemeal breadcrumbs
- 40g/⅓ cup grated mozzarella cheese
- 40g/⅓ cup grated cheddar cheese

Serve with large side salad and fresh brown rolls.

Method

1. Line a sided baking sheet with parchment paper. Rub each mushroom with a bit of olive oil and set them on the sheet, stalk side up.

2. Over a medium-high heat, add the oil and onions to a pan. Sauté for 3–4 minutes, then add the courgette, red pepper and tomatoes. Cook until the courgette is getting soft and the onions are translucent. Add the garlic, followed by the spinach.

3. Preheat your oven to 190°C/375°F (fan 170°C /325°F) or gas mark 5.

4. Once the spinach wilts, remove the pan from the heat and add the rest of the ingredients, excluding the cheese. Stir to combine.

5. Fill each mushroom evenly with the mixture.

6. Bake in the oven for about 10–15 minutes. Mix the two grated cheeses together and top each mushroom with about 1 tbsp of cheese and continue baking for another 10 to 12 minutes, or until the cheese is just beginning to get golden on top.

7. Serve with a large green salad and fresh brown rolls.

NUTRITION INFORMATION
Amount per serving

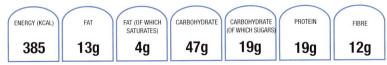

ENERGY (KCAL)	FAT	FAT (OF WHICH SATURATES)	CARBOHYDRATE	CARBOHYDRATE (OF WHICH SUGARS)	PROTEIN	FIBRE
385	13g	4g	47g	19g	19g	12g

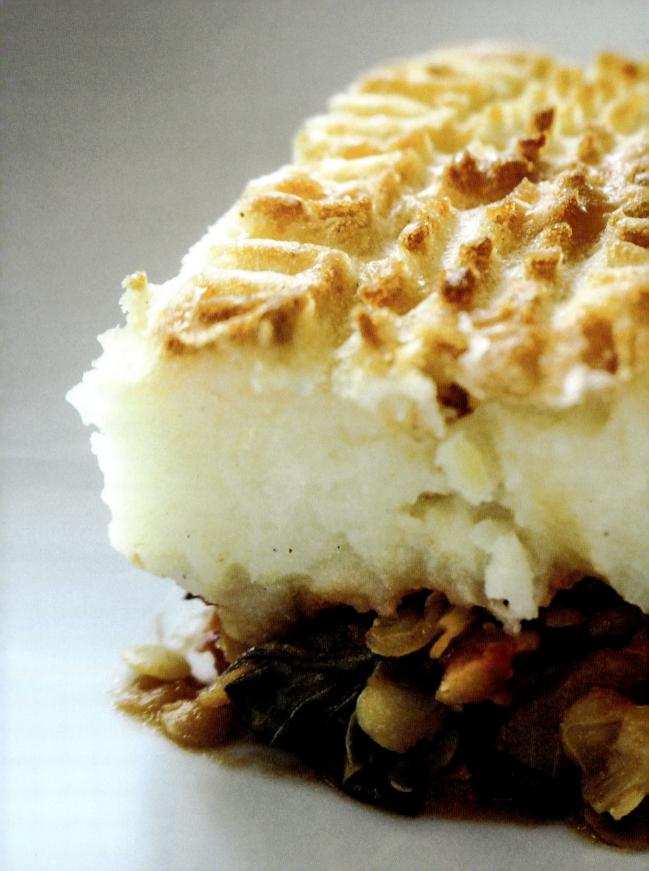

Vegetable and red lentil pie

🍽 **Serves:** 6 ⏱ **Prep time:** 20 mins ♨ **Cooking time:** 1 hour 30 mins

Ingredients

- 2 tbsp. olive oil
- 2 onions, chopped
- 2 garlic cloves, finely chopped
- 2 carrots, chopped into small cubes
- 300g/11oz piece of turnip or swede, chopped into small cubes
- 125g/1²/₃ cups red dried lentils
- 400g/14oz tin plum tomatoes
- 1 tbsp. sun-dried tomato paste
- 350ml/1½ cups vegetable stock
- Large handful spinach leaves
- 6 potatoes, peeled and cut into large chunks
- 30g/2 tbsp. butter
- 5 tbsp. semi-skimmed/skimmed milk
- Freshly ground black pepper
- 100g/1 cup low-fat cheddar cheese, coarsely grated

Method

1. Heat 1 tbsp. of the oil in a large, non-stick pan. Add the onions and garlic and fry for 8–10 minutes over a medium-high heat or until starting to turn golden, stirring occasionally.

2. Pour the remaining tbsp. of oil into the pan, tip in the carrots and swede, and fry for 3 minutes.

3. Reduce the heat to medium. Stir in the lentils, tomatoes, sun-dried tomato paste and stock. Season and simmer, covered, for 35–40 minutes over a low heat, until the carrots, swede and lentils are tender.

4. Remove from the heat, stir in the spinach and let it wilt. Pour the mixture into the baking dish. Leave to cool. Preheat the oven to 200°C/400°F (fan 180⁰C/400⁰F) or gas mark 6.

5. Put the potatoes into a large pan and cover with cold water. Bring to the boil and simmer for 15–20 minutes or until tender. Drain well.

6. Put the butter and milk in the pan and warm through over a low heat. Remove from the heat, return the potatoes to the pan, and mash with the milk and butter, then whisk until smooth. Season with pepper, then stir in the cheese.

7. Spread the mash over the filling and bake for 30–40 minutes until golden and bubbling.

NUTRITION INFORMATION
Amount per serving

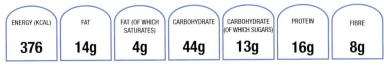

ENERGY (KCAL)	FAT	FAT (OF WHICH SATURATES)	CARBOHYDRATE	CARBOHYDRATE (OF WHICH SUGARS)	PROTEIN	FIBRE
376	14g	4g	44g	13g	16g	8g

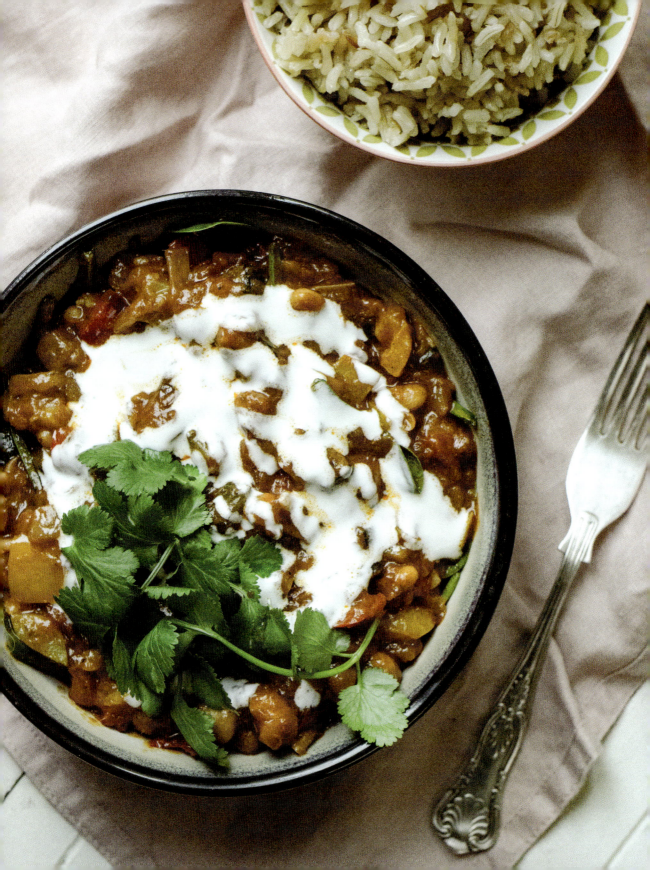

Vegetable jalfrezi

🍽 **Serves:** 4 ⏱ **Prep time:** 20 mins 🍵 **Cooking time:** 30 mins

Ingredients

- 1 tbsp. sunflower oil
- 2 large onions, sliced
- 2–3 green chilli peppers, chopped
- 3 cloves garlic, crushed
- 2 tbsp. ginger, finely grated
- 5 tomatoes, skinned and chopped, or
  1 x 400g/14oz tin of chopped tomatoes
- 2 peppers, chopped
- 1 courgette, chopped
- Approx. 100ml/½ cup stock or water
- 1 tin chickpeas or mixed beans, drained
- Handful baby leaf spinach
- 2 tbsp. fresh coriander
- 100ml/½ cup natural yogurt

Spice mix:
- 2 tsp. ground turmeric
- 2 tsp. ground cumin
- 2 tsp. ground coriander
- 1 tsp. ground cloves
- Freshly ground black pepper
- 1 cinnamon stick

Method

1. Heat the oil in a large pan. Add the onion and fry until beginning to turn golden.

2. Add the chillies, garlic and ginger. Cook for 3–4 minutes.

3. Add the spice mix and cook for another minute. Then add the tomatoes, peppers and courgette.

4. Stir well and add the stock or water.

5. Add chickpeas/beans, cover the pan and cook for about 20 minutes on a gentle heat.

6. Remove the cinnamon stick. Stir in the spinach, yogurt and coriander just before serving.

NUTRITION INFORMATION
Amount per serving

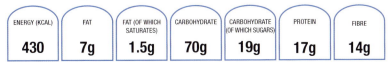

ENERGY (KCAL)	FAT	FAT (OF WHICH SATURATES)	CARBOHYDRATE	CARBOHYDRATE (OF WHICH SUGARS)	PROTEIN	FIBRE
430	7g	1.5g	70g	19g	17g	14g

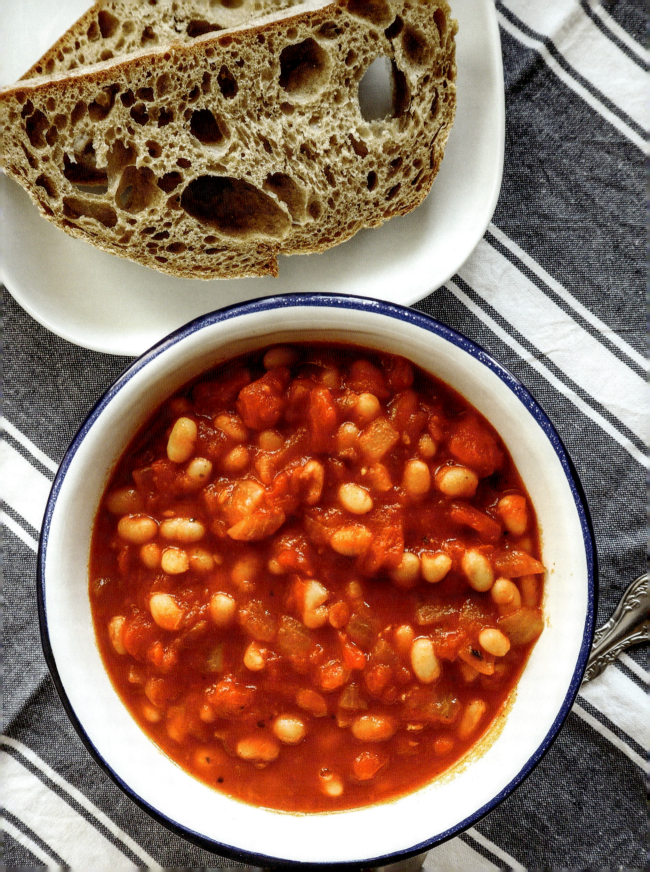

Butter bean stew

Serves: 2 **Prep time:** 5 mins **Cooking time:** 20 mins

Ingredients

- 1 onion, chopped
- 2 cloves garlic, finely chopped
- 1 tsp. olive oil
- 1 x 400g/14oz tin butter beans, drained
- 1 x 400g/14oz tin chopped tomatoes
- 3–4 tsp. smoked paprika
- Freshly ground black pepper
- Crusty bread

Method

1. In a saucepan, cook the chopped onion and garlic in olive oil until soft.

2. Drain and rinse the butter beans and add to the pot with the chopped tomatoes.

3. Add the smoked paprika and stir through.

4. Cover and simmer for 10 minutes – the sauce should reduce down to a thick stew consistency.

5. Add freshly ground black pepper to taste. Divide into two bowls and serve with crusty bread to mop up the juices.

NUTRITION INFORMATION
Amount per serving

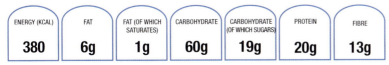

ENERGY (KCAL)	FAT	FAT (OF WHICH SATURATES)	CARBOHYDRATE	CARBOHYDRATE (OF WHICH SUGARS)	PROTEIN	FIBRE
380	6g	1g	60g	19g	20g	13g

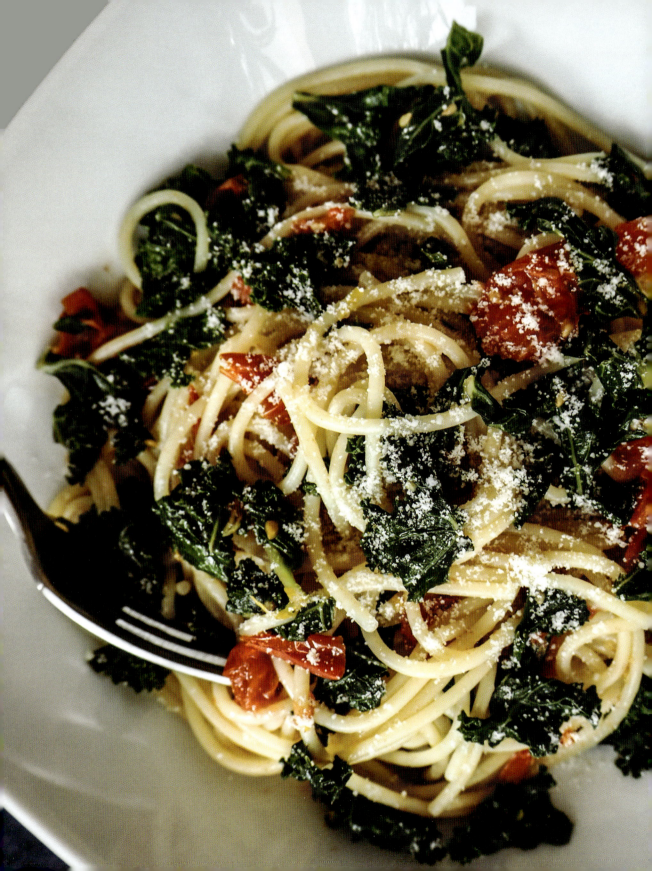

Kale, tomato and lemon spaghetti

🍽 **Serves:** 4 ⏱ **Prep time:** 5 mins 🍲 **Cooking time:** 30 mins

Ingredients

- 250g/9oz wholewheat spaghetti
- 300g/1½ cups cherry tomatoes
- Zest of ½ a lemon
- Juice of ½ a lemon
- 40ml/1½oz olive oil
- 600ml/2½ cups boiling water
- 1 bag of chopped kale (around 150–200g/5–7oz)
- 40g/⅓ cup grated parmesan cheese

Method

1. Roughly chop the tomatoes and add to the pan with the olive oil. Grate the zest from the lemon half, making sure just to get the outer layer and not the bitter white part underneath. Add to the pan.

2. Bring 600ml/2½ cups water to the boil in a large pot. Put a lid on the pan and bring to the boil. When it is boiling, remove the lid, add the spaghetti and simmer on a high heat until the spaghetti is cooked (6–10 minutes), turning the pasta frequently with a tongs to ensure even cooking.

3. Remove any tough stems from the kale and tear the leaves. When the pasta is nearly cooked add the kale, tomatoes, lemon juice and zest. Simmer for 2 more minutes, turning the kale in the other ingredients. The kale will seem very bulky when added to the pot (hence the need for a big pot) but will very quickly reduce down as it heats.

4. Once almost all the water has evaporated, you will be left with a nice thick sauce coating the spaghetti.

5. Divide into 4 bowls and sprinkle with parmesan.

NUTRITION INFORMATION
Amount per serving

ENERGY (KCAL)	FAT	FAT (OF WHICH SATURATES)	CARBOHYDRATE	CARBOHYDRATE (OF WHICH SUGARS)	PROTEIN	SALT	FIBRE
393	16g	3.8g	42g	5.8g	10g	0.23g	14g

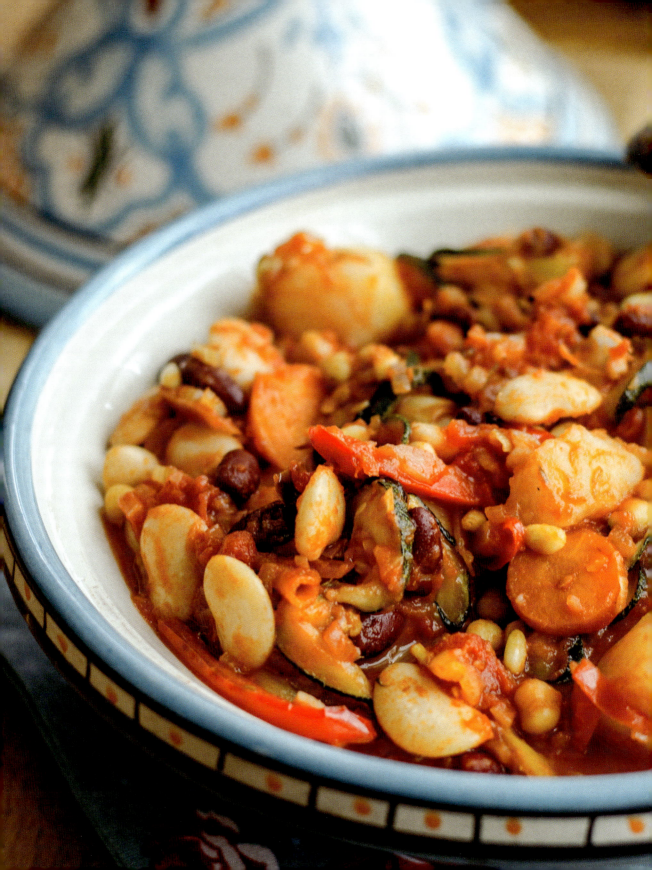

Vegetarian casserole

🍽 **Serves:** 4 ⏱ **Prep time:** 20 mins 🍵 **Cooking time:** 40 mins

Ingredients

- 1 red pepper, chopped
- 1 yellow pepper, chopped
- 1 carrot, diced
- 1 courgette, diced
- 1 tbsp. olive oil
- 600g/1¼lb baby potatoes (allow 5 per person)
- 1 red onion, sliced
- 1 fennel bulb, sliced
- 4 cloves garlic, chopped
- 2 x 400g/14oz tins plum tomatoes
- 2 tbsp. tomato puree
- 1 tsp. dried oregano
- 1 x 400g/14oz tin butter beans or mixed beans, drained
- 1 x 400g/14oz tin kidney beans, drained
- ½ tin of chickpeas, drained
- 1 tsp. brown sugar
- Freshly ground black pepper for seasoning
- 50g/¹/₃ cup pine nuts

Method

1. Preheat the oven to 200°C/400°F (fan 180°C/350°F) or gas mark 6. Toss the peppers, courgette and carrots with the olive oil and roast in the oven. Set aside when ready. Boil the potatoes until almost fully cooked, strain and set aside.

2. While the vegetables are roasting, slice the onion and fennel thinly and chop the garlic. Sweat these ingredients together in a little olive oil for 15 minutes, stirring occasionally.

3. Add the chopped tomatoes, tomato puree and dried oregano. Cook for 20–30 minutes on a low heat until the sauce has thickened.

4. Stir in the roast vegetables, kidney beans, butter beans, chickpeas and baby potatoes. Season with some pepper. Add a pinch of brown sugar. Simmer for a further 5 minutes.

5. Sprinkle with pine nuts and serve.

NUTRITION INFORMATION
Amount per serving

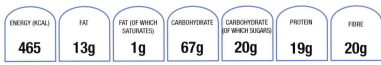

ENERGY (KCAL)	FAT	FAT (OF WHICH SATURATES)	CARBOHYDRATE	CARBOHYDRATE (OF WHICH SUGARS)	PROTEIN	FIBRE
465	13g	1g	67g	20g	19g	20g

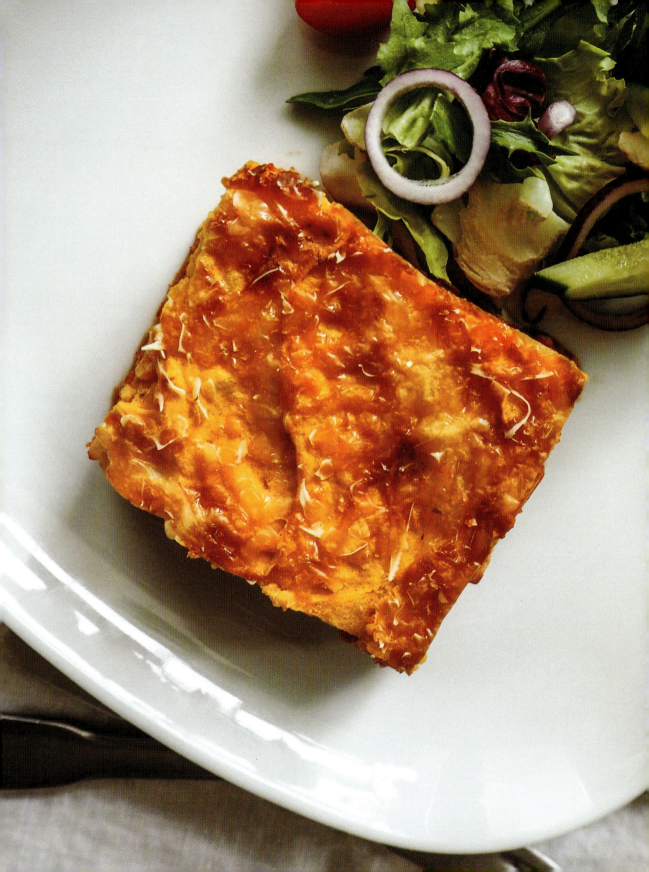

Quorn pie

Serves: 4 · Prep time: 15 mins · Cooking time: 1 hour–1 hour 10 mins

Ingredients

- 400g/14oz potatoes, peeled and cut into even cubes
- 400g/14oz sweet potatoes, peeled and cut into even cubes
- 1 tbsp. olive oil
- 1 small onion, finely chopped
- 2 cloves garlic, chopped
- 1 stick of celery, chopped
- 1 carrot, peeled and chopped
- 1 tbsp. chopped rosemary leaves
- 350g/12oz packet of Quorn mince
- 1 tbsp. plain flour
- 700g/1½lb jar of passata
- 220g/8oz tin of butter beans, drained
- Pepper to season
- 80g/¾ cup of low-fat cheddar cheese, grated

Method

1. Bring a large saucepan of water to the boil and add the chunks of potato and sweet potato. Cover and boil until soft, roughly 20 minutes. Drain, mash and season with pepper.

2. Meanwhile preheat the oven to 190°C/375°F (fan 170°C /325°F) or gas mark 5.

3. Heat a non-stick pan and add the oil. Gently fry the garlic, onion, celery, carrot and rosemary for 5–8 minutes to soften.

4. Next, stir in the mince and flour. Pour in the passata and allow to simmer for 5 minutes.

5. Stir in the butter beans and season with pepper.

6. Transfer the mince mixture to a large ovenproof dish. Top with the mash and spread evenly with a fork. Sprinkle with the grated cheese and place in the preheated oven.

7. Bake for 40–45 minutes until cooked through and bubbling.

NUTRITION INFORMATION
Amount per serving

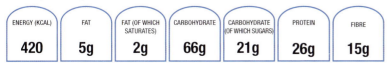

ENERGY (KCAL)	FAT	FAT (OF WHICH SATURATES)	CARBOHYDRATE	CARBOHYDRATE (OF WHICH SUGARS)	PROTEIN	FIBRE
420	5g	2g	66g	21g	26g	15g

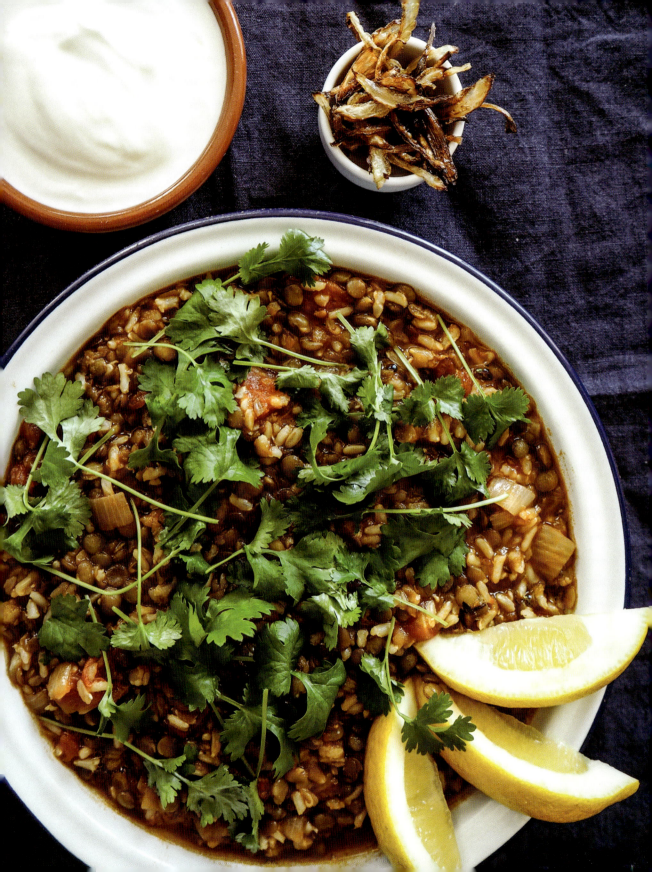

Spicy rice and lentil one-pot

🍽 **Serves:** 8 ⏱ **Prep time:** 10 mins 🍲 **Cooking time:** 50 mins

Ingredients

- 1 tbsp. olive oil
- 1 large onion, peeled and chopped
- 2 tsp. cumin seeds
- 2 tsp. coriander seeds
- ½ tsp. of black peppercorns
- 2 garlic cloves, peeled and chopped
- 500g/2½ cups green lentils
- 300g/1⅓ cups wholegrain rice
- 3 tins of chopped tomatoes
- 1000ml/4¼ cups vegetable stock

Garnish:
- 1 tbsp. olive oil
- 1 large onion, thinly sliced
- 1 lemon cut into wedges
- Coriander sprigs
- Low-fat Greek-style yogurt

Method

1. Heat the oil in a large pan, add the onion and fry for 5 minutes until lightly browned. Meanwhile crush the cumin, coriander seeds and peppercorns (using a pestle and mortar) and add these plus the garlic to the pan. Fry for 2 minutes, add the lentils and the rice, and then stir.

2. Add the tomatoes and stock and bring to the boil.

3. Cover and simmer for 40 minutes until the lentils are tender.

4. To make the garnish, heat the oil in a frying pan, add the sliced onion and fry over a high heat for 5 minutes until crisp. Drain on kitchen paper and spoon the onion over the lentil mixture and garnish with lemon wedges and coriander. Serve with a dollop of low-fat Greek-style yogurt.

NUTRITION INFORMATION
Amount per serving

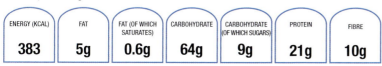

ENERGY (KCAL)	FAT	FAT (OF WHICH SATURATES)	CARBOHYDRATE	CARBOHYDRATE (OF WHICH SUGARS)	PROTEIN	FIBRE
383	5g	0.6g	64g	9g	21g	10g

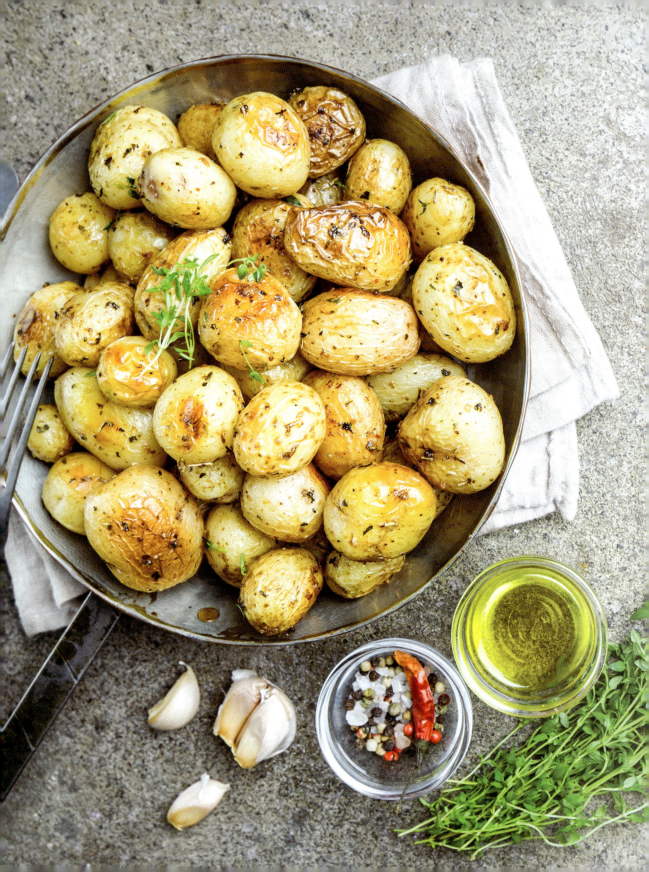

Side dishes

Champ mash potato

Mustard mash

Roast garlic baby potatoes

Spicy potato wedges

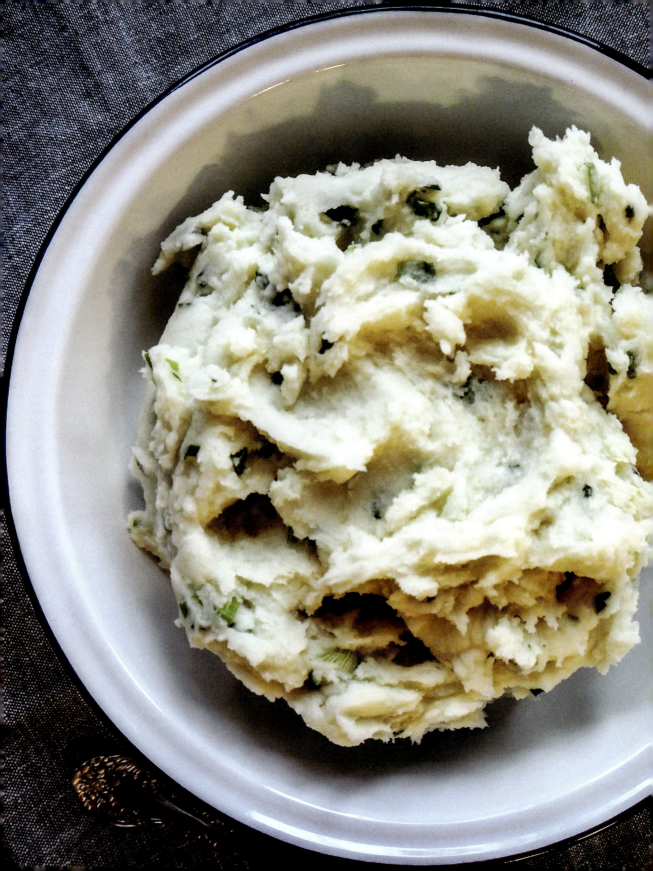

Champm mash potato

🍽 **Serves:** 4 ⏱ **Prep time:** 10 mins 🍲 **Cooking time:** 30 mins

Ingredients

- 600g/1¼lb potatoes, peeled and cut in even chunks
- 100ml/½ cup semi-skimmed milk, approximately
- 15g/1 tbsp. butter
- 4 spring onions, chopped
- Seasoning

Method

1. Boil the potatoes until cooked.

2. Drain and mash.

3. Warm the milk and stir into the potatoes and season.

4. Cook the spring onions gently in the butter and beat into the potatoes.

NUTRITION INFORMATION
Amount per serving

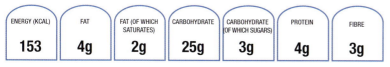

ENERGY (KCAL)	FAT	FAT (OF WHICH SATURATES)	CARBOHYDRATE	CARBOHYDRATE (OF WHICH SUGARS)	PROTEIN	FIBRE
153	4g	2g	25g	3g	4g	3g

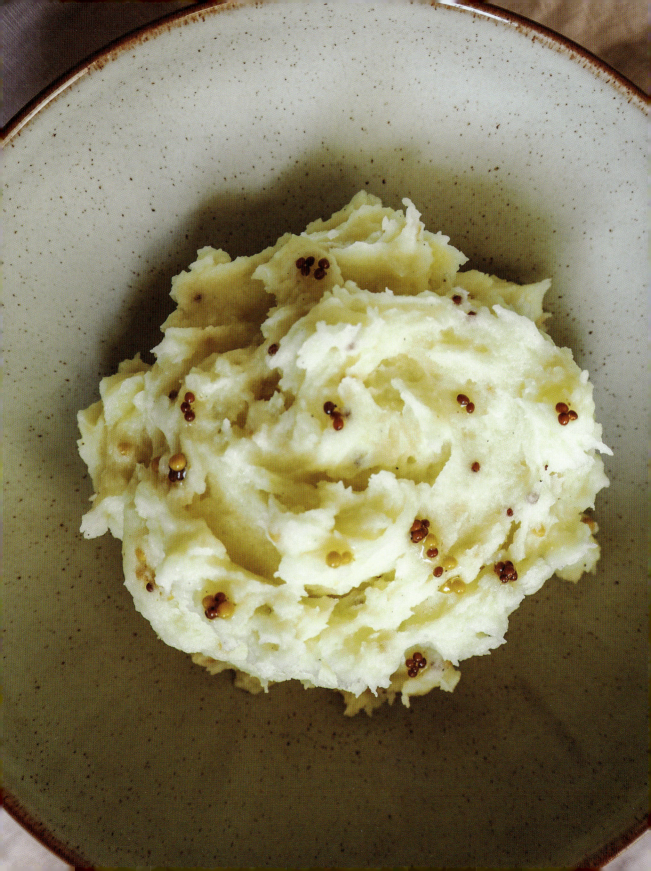

Mustard mash

🍽 **Serves:** 4 ⏱ **Prep time:** 10 mins 🍲 **Cooking time:** 20 mins

Ingredients

- 600g/1¼lb new potatoes, washed and halved
- 1 tbsp. olive oil
- 3 tsp. wholegrain mustard

Method

1. Boil the potatoes until cooked.

2. Drain the water off the potatoes. Mix the olive oil and mustard with the potatoes and then mash.

NUTRITION INFORMATION
Amount per serving

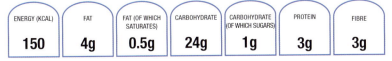

ENERGY (KCAL)	FAT	FAT (OF WHICH SATURATES)	CARBOHYDRATE	CARBOHYDRATE (OF WHICH SUGARS)	PROTEIN	FIBRE
150	4g	0.5g	24g	1g	3g	3g

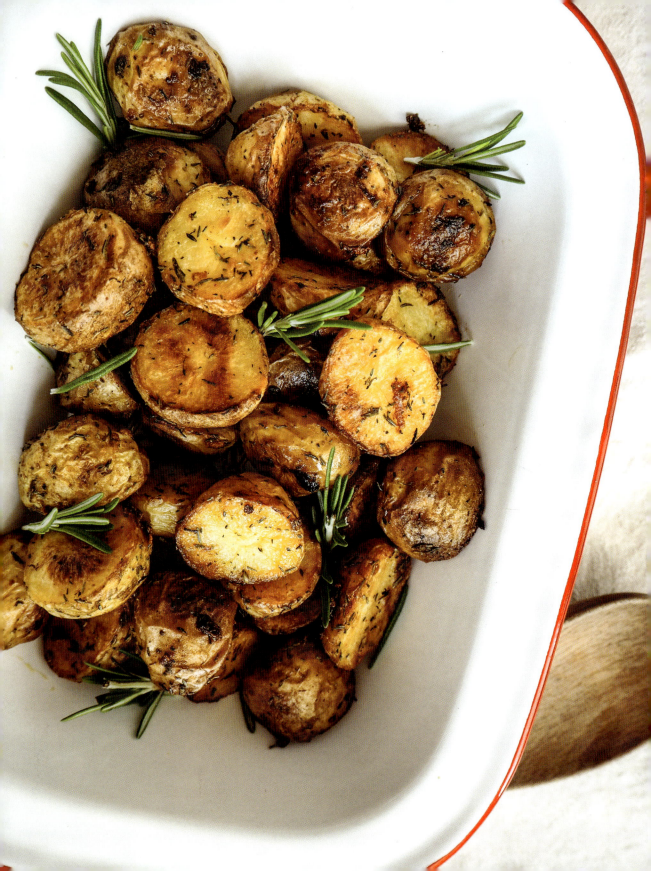

Roast garlic baby potatoes

🍽 **Serves:** 4 ⏱ **Prep time:** 10 mins 🍲 **Cooking time:** 30 mins

Ingredients

- 800g/1¾lb baby potatoes
- 2 tbsp. olive oil
- 2 tbsp. fresh rosemary, finely chopped
- 2–3 cloves garlic, chopped
- Freshly ground black pepper

Method

1. Rinse the baby potatoes and chop in half.

2. Place in a roasting dish and use enough olive oil to coat the potatoes lightly (2 tbsp.).

3. Stir in the chopped garlic and season with rosemary and freshly ground black pepper.

4. Roast in the oven for 25–35 minutes at 180°C/350°F (fan 160°C/320°F) or gas mark 4.

NUTRITION INFORMATION
Amount per serving

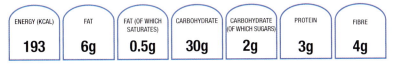

ENERGY (KCAL)	FAT	FAT (OF WHICH SATURATES)	CARBOHYDRATE	CARBOHYDRATE (OF WHICH SUGARS)	PROTEIN	FIBRE
193	6g	0.5g	30g	2g	3g	4g

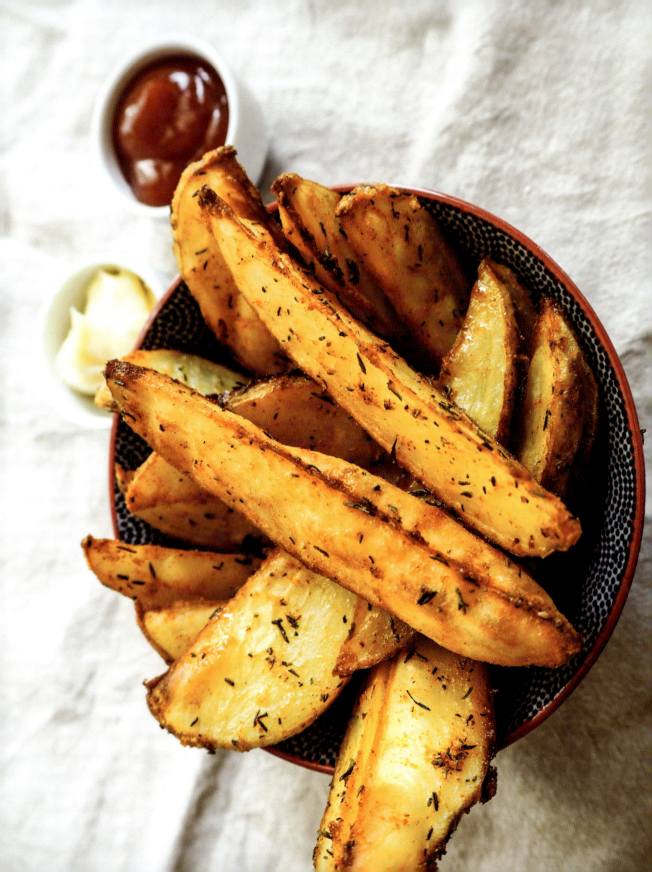

Spicy potato wedges

⟨Ⓘ⟩ Serves: 4 ⏱ **Prep time:** 10 mins ♨ **Cooking time:** 30 mins

Ingredients

- 4 large potatoes
- 2 tbsp. olive/sunflower/rapeseed oil
- Salt and freshly ground black pepper
- 1–2 tsp. Cajun seasoning

Method

1. Scrub the potatoes well and cut into wedges.

2. Rinse, dry and put on a baking tray.

3. Toss in oil and add salt, pepper and Cajun seasoning.

NUTRITION INFORMATION
Amount per serving

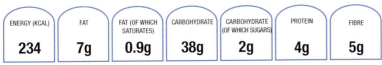

ENERGY (KCAL)	FAT	FAT (OF WHICH SATURATES)	CARBOHYDRATE	CARBOHYDRATE (OF WHICH SUGARS)	PROTEIN	FIBRE
234	7g	0.9g	38g	2g	4g	5g

About the authors

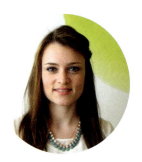

Dr Éadaoin Ní Bhuachalla PhD RD

Dr Éadaoin Ní Bhuachalla graduated with an honours degree in Human Nutrition and Dietetics from Dublin Institute of Technology/Trinity College Dublin in 2013. Following this, she joined Dr Aoife Ryan's research team in University College Cork and Mercy University Hospital. There, her research and publications focused on the identification, impact and treatment of malnutrition in the oncology setting, as well as the role of nutrition in cancer prevention. Éadaoin has co-authored nutritional resources for patients suffering from cancer-induced weight loss that include high-protein, high-calorie recipes tailored to meet their nutritional needs. To date, 29,000 copies of these resources have been printed and distributed to more than 74 health care locations nationwide free of charge. In 2015, the *Good Nutrition for Cancer Recovery* cookbook received an Irish Health Care Award for the Best Patient Lifestyle Education Initiative. Éadaoin was awarded her PhD in 2017 under the supervision of Dr Aoife Ryan and Dr Derek Power in University College Cork. In 2018, Éadaoin joined the Health Service Executive, where she now works as a Senior Primary Care Dietitian. She is a CORU Registered Dietitian in Ireland.

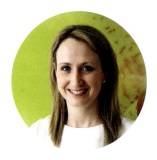

Dr Aoife Ryan PhD RD

Dr Aoife Ryan graduated with an honours degree in Human Nutrition and Dietetics from Trinity College Dublin/Dublin Institute of Technology in 2000 and was the recipient of a Trinity College Gold Medal. She initially worked as a dietitian at St James's Hospital for eight years in the area of surgical oncology, during which time she completed her PhD (2008) at Trinity College Dublin under the supervision of Prof. John Reynolds on the topic of nutrition and upper gastrointestinal cancer. In 2008 she was appointed Assistant Professor of Nutrition and Dietetics at New York University. She returned to Ireland and joined the academic staff of University College Cork in 2011, where she is now a senior lecturer in nutrition and dietetics. Aoife is a CORU Registered Dietitian in Ireland and also holds a Postgraduate Diploma in Teaching & Learning in Higher Education. Aoife runs an active research programme on nutrition and cancer at University College Cork. She has previously been awarded INDI Research Dietitian of the Year and both the Julie Wallace Medal and Cuthbertson Medal from the Nutrition Society. Aoife has published many scientific journal articles and four cookbooks for cancer patients which have all been professionally endorsed and have received a number of awards.

With a rising tide of misinformation on nutrition and cancer in the media and online, Éadaoin and Aoife decided to partner with Breakthrough Cancer Research to write this book as an evidence-based resource for individuals who wish to eat a healthier diet to lower their risk of cancer. This book is also suitable for cancer patients entering the survivorship phase of their illness who have been advised to follow a healthy-eating diet.

Acknowledgements

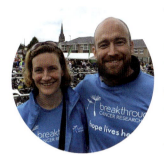

The authors would like to acknowledge the key roles played by Ms Orla Dolan and Mr Eoghan O'Sullivan and colleagues in Breakthrough Cancer Research for making the idea of this book come to life through their incredible support and encouragement (www.breakthroughcancerresearch.ie).

The authors would also like to acknowledge culinary lecturers Jane Healy and Anne O'Connor from Cork Institute of Technology, who helped with recipe development and editing of this book. They would also like to acknowledge the contribution of Dr Jackie Lyons in the introductory text.

The authors are also grateful to Anna Twomey for her assistance with the recipe analysis.

The authors are also hugely grateful to Marta and Jacub Miklinska, who performed the food styling and food photography used in this book.

The authors would also like to thank Kasia Uszczynska for all her hard work on the layout and design of this book.

The authors would also like to acknowledge the dietitians, chefs, cooks, cancer experts and nutritionists who contributed recipes to this book:

Bean chilli - Celene Sands
Butter bean stew - Dr Con Murphy
Butternut squash, chickpea and spinach curry - Lorraine Fitzmaurice
Chicken fajita stuffed peppers - Gemma Fagan
Chicken, bean and kale stew - Sarah Browne
Chickpea and mango salad - Derval O'Rourke
Chilli con carne - Gemma Fagan
Courgette and feta fritters - Tracey Kelly
Fish pie - Georgina Campbell
Fisherman's stew - Joanne McEldowney
Fruity chicken tagine - Philomena Flood
Grilled chicken with green lentil dahl - Fiona Dwyer
Grilled lemon-scented salmon - Odran Lawlor
Kale, tomato and lemon spaghetti - Dr Con Murphy
Lamb tagine - Sheila Sugrue
Millet, sweet potato and cashew burgers - Lorraine Fitzmaurice
Minestrone - Fiona Dwyer
Pink tabbouleh salad - Sarah Browne

Pitta with chicken, carrot and coriander salad - Liz Moore
Quinoa with roasted vegetables and feta - Lorraine Fitzmaurice
Quorn pie - Arún Fenton
Rainbow salad - WCRF
Red lentil and tomato soup - Karina Carroll
Roast garlic baby potatoes - Catherine Shortall
Roast squash, bean and kale salad - Sarah Browne
Salmon and pasta salad - Ellen Barrett
Salmon linguine - Joanne McEldowney
Seared haddock with horseradish aioli - Croí Galway
Soda bread - WCRF
Spicy chicken pitta - Derval O'Rourke
Spicy rice and lentil one-pot - Arún Fenton
Sweet and sour pork - WCRF
Tandoori chicken fillet burger - Croí Galway
Three-grain salad - Derval O'Rourke
Tomato and cannellini bean soup - Derval O'Rourke
Warm shredded chicken and chilli salad - Tracey Kelly

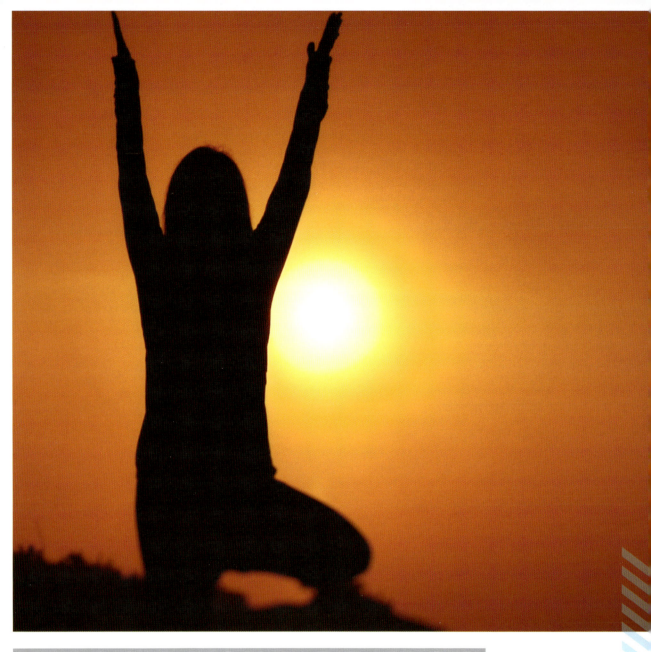

HELP MORE PEOPLE LIVE LONGER

When you fund us, you are supporting the frontline of cancer research.

Our work has led to 300 new discoveries on cancer understanding and treatment to date and helped produce evidence-based resources like the recipes in our books. Our researchers are leading the world in developing treatments and approaches that will get us to 100% survival for 100% of all cancers sooner. Your help is vital.

It will get innovative treatments from the lab to patients faster.

Please donate at breakthroughcancerresearch.ie today
Let's **#makemoresurvivors**

breakthroug
CANCER RESEARC

breakthrough
CANCER RESEARCH

The production of this book would not
have been possible without the support of
Breakthrough Cancer Research.

First published in 2020 by Atrium
Atrium is an imprint of
Cork University Press
Boole Library
University College Cork
Cork
T12 ND89
Ireland

Library of Congress Control Number: 2020939352

Distribution in the USA Longleaf Services, Chapel Hill, NC, USA

ISBN 9781782054252
Book design and typesetting by Kasia Uszczynska
Printed in Malta by Gutenberg Press

Cover image: shutterstock.com

Index

A

almonds
- butter bean and almond dip, 157
- crunchy tossed salad, 87
- pasta with turkey, almond and rocket, 223
- rainbow salad, 105
- spicy chicken pitta, 137

apples
- healthy coleslaw, 169
- rainbow salad, 105
- spiced pork tray bake, 197

apricots
- fruity chicken tagine, 215
- rainbow salad, 105

asparagus
- salmon linguine, 253

aubergine
- aubergine and coriander dip, 167
- ratatouille, 279

avocado
- crunchy tossed salad, 87
- easy guacamole, 159
- glazed salmon, 243
- Mexican beans on toast, 121
- quick salad with berries, 99

B

baby corn *see* sweetcorn

baked beans
- baked potato with baked beans, 125
- bean chilli, 265

baked cod with a vine tomato topping, 235

baked hake/cod with a herb crust, 259

baked potatoes
- with baked beans, 125
- with bean chilli, 125, 265
- with beef chilli, 125, 185
- with chicken, spring onion and cream cheese, 125
- with chunky salsa and cheese, 125, 173
- with salmon, 125
- with tuna and sweetcorn, 125

basil
- creamy chicken and tomato bake, 227
- Italian salad, 93
- Mediterranean fish tray bake, 249
- millet, sweet potato and cashew burgers, 275
- minestrone soup, 61
- pasta with turkey, almond and rocket, 223
- quinoa with roasted vegetables and feta, 95
- salmon and pasta salad, 91
- spaghetti bolognese, 195
- spicy Italian cod, 261
- tomato and cannellini bean soup, 71

bean chilli, 265

bean sprouts
- crunchy tossed salad, 87
- egg-fried rice, 271

beans *see* baked beans; black beans; butter beans; cannellini beans; chickpeas; green beans; kidney beans; mixed beans; pinto beans

beef
- beef burgers, 179
- beef stew, 181
- beef stroganoff, 183
- chilli con carne, 185
- healthy lasagne, 191
- Italian meatballs with pasta, 187
- shepherd's pie, 193
- spaghetti bolognese, 195
- steak with salsa verde, 199

beetroot
- healthy coleslaw, 169
- pink tabbouleh salad, 107

black beans: Mexican beans on toast, 121

Brazil nuts: pitta with chicken, carrot and coriander salad, 141

breads
- brown bread with seeds, 83
- oat bread, 79
- soda bread, 81

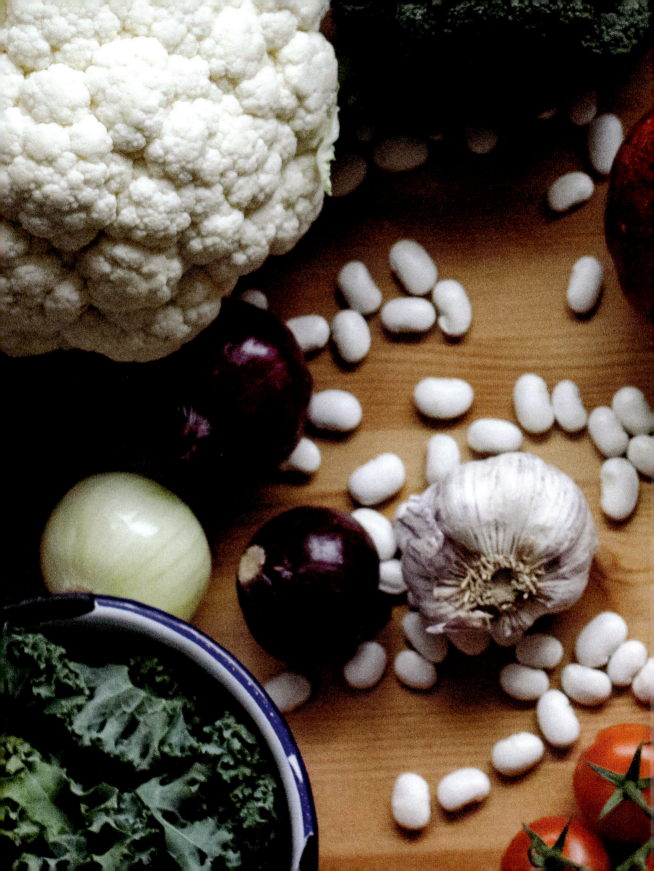

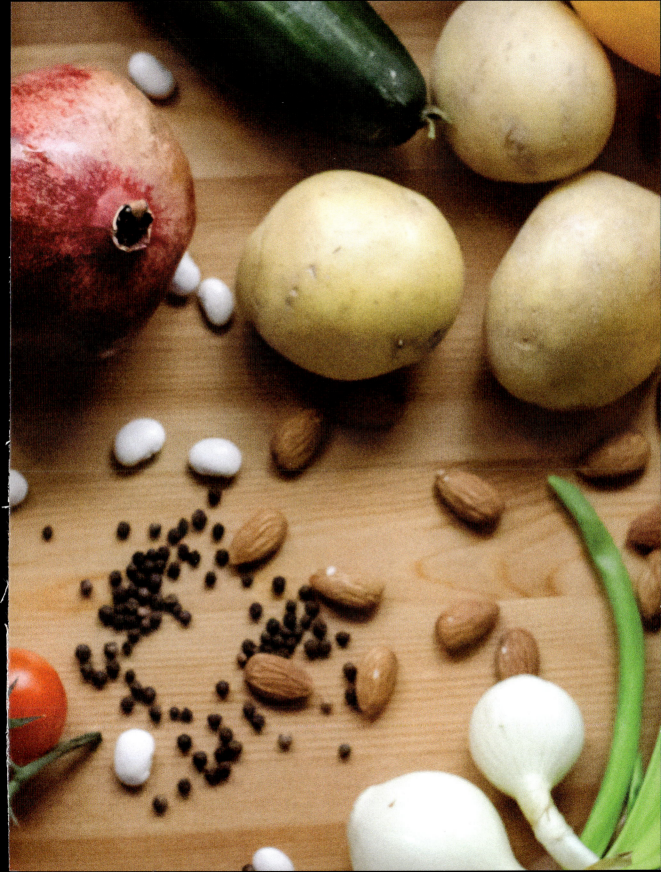

Notes